About the NCCN Guidelines for Patients®

AF702263

NCCN National Comprehensive Cancer Network®

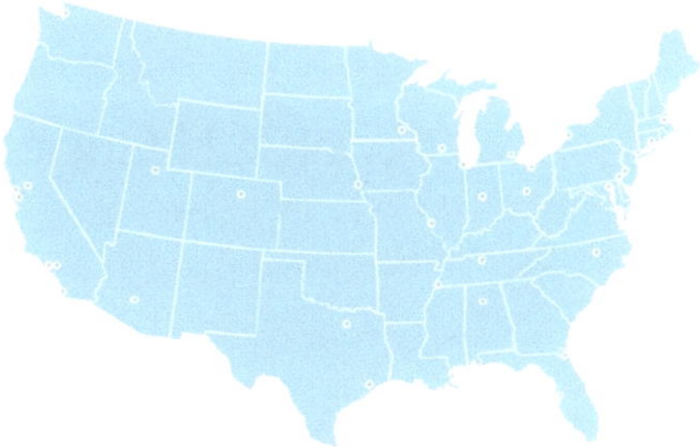

Did you know that top cancer centers across the United States work together to improve cancer care? This alliance of leading cancer centers is called the National Comprehensive Cancer Network® (NCCN®).

Cancer care is always changing. NCCN develops evidence-based cancer care recommendations used by health care providers worldwide. These frequently updated recommendations are the NCCN Clinical Practice Guidelines in Oncology (NCCN Guidelines®). The NCCN Guidelines for Patients plainly explain these expert recommendations for people with cancer and caregivers.

These NCCN Guidelines for Patients are based on the NCCN Clinical Practice Guidelines in Oncology (NCCN Guidelines®) for Primary Cutaneous Lymphomas Version 3.2024 – August 22, 2024.

View the NCCN Guidelines for Patients free online
NCCN.org/patientguidelines

Find an NCCN Cancer Center near you
NCCN.org/cancercenters

Connect with us

Supporters

NATIONAL COMPREHENSIVE CANCER NETWORK®
NCCN FOUNDATION
Guiding Treatment. Changing Lives.

NCCN Guidelines for Patients are supported by funding from the NCCN Foundation®

NCCN independently adapts, updates, and hosts the NCCN Guidelines for Patients. Our corporate supporters do not participate in the development of the NCCN Guidelines for Patients and are not responsible for the content and recommendations contained therein.

To make a gift or learn more, visit online or email

NCCNFoundation.org/donate

PatientGuidelines@NCCN.org

Contents

© 2024 National Comprehensive Cancer Network, Inc. All rights reserved. NCCN Guidelines for Patients and illustrations herein may not be reproduced in any form for any purpose without the express written permission of NCCN. No one, including doctors or patients, may use the NCCN Guidelines for Patients for any commercial purpose and may not claim, represent, or imply that the NCCN Guidelines for Patients that have been modified in any manner are derived from, based on, related to, or arise out of the NCCN Guidelines for Patients. The NCCN Guidelines are a work in progress that may be redefined as often as new significant data become available. NCCN makes no warranties of any kind whatsoever regarding its content, use, or application and disclaims any responsibility for its application or use in any way.

NCCN Foundation seeks to support the millions of patients and their families affected by a cancer diagnosis by funding and distributing NCCN Guidelines for Patients. NCCN Foundation is also committed to advancing cancer treatment by funding the nation's promising doctors at the center of innovation in cancer research. For more details and the full library of patient and caregiver resources, visit NCCN.org/patients.

National Comprehensive Cancer Network (NCCN) and NCCN Foundation
3025 Chemical Road, Suite 100, Plymouth Meeting, PA 19462 USA

1

CTCL basics

Cutaneous T-cell lymphoma (CTCL) develops when T cell lymphocytes grow abnormally in the skin. A lymphocyte is a type of white blood cell that helps fight and prevent infection. CTCL can grow in other areas of the body such as the blood and lymph nodes. CTCL is not skin cancer.

Lymphatic system

Lymphoma is the most common type of blood cancer. It affects the lymphatic system. The lymphatic or lymph system is a major part of the body's immune system. It is a germ-fighting network of tissues and organs that includes the bone marrow, spleen, thymus, lymph nodes, and lymphatic vessels.

Lymphatic vessels are a network of thin tubes that carry lymphatic fluid (lymph) and white blood cells into all the tissues of the body. Lymph gives cells water and food. White blood cells, such as lymphocytes, help fight infection and disease.

Lymphatic system

The lymphatic system is part of your immune system. It includes the bone marrow, spleen, thymus, lymph nodes, and lymphatic vessels.

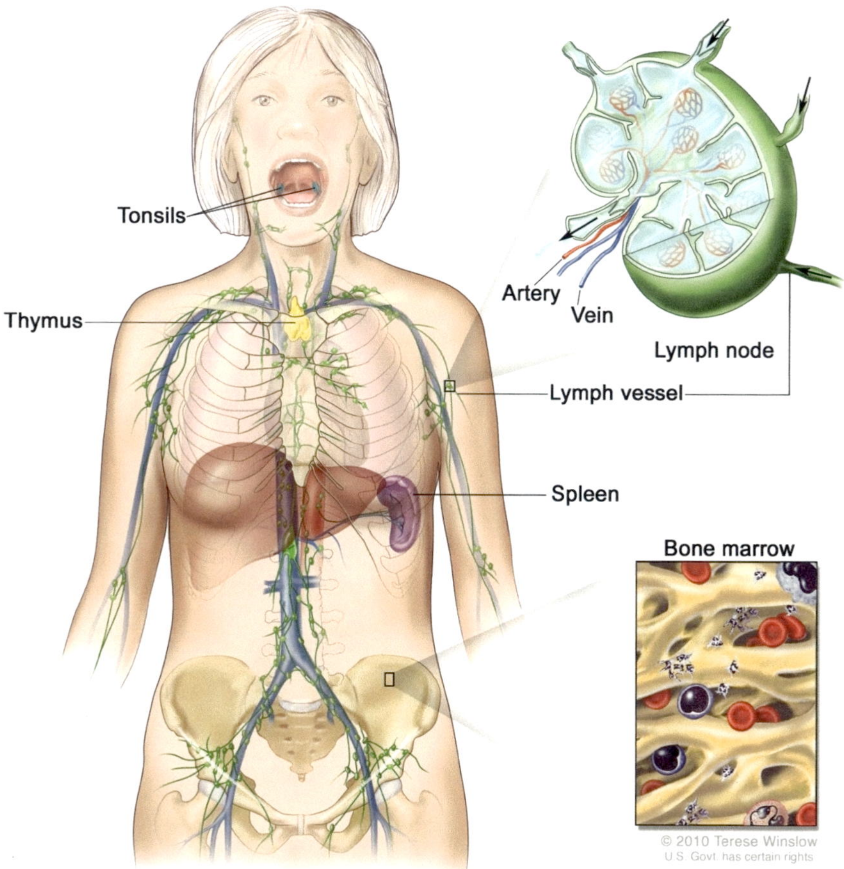

As lymph travels throughout your body, it passes through hundreds of small bean-shaped structures called lymph nodes. Lymph nodes make immune cells that help the body fight infection. They also filter the lymph fluid and remove foreign material such as bacteria and cancer cells.

Lymphocytes

Non-Hodgkin lymphoma (NHL) is a cancer of lymphocytes. A lymphocyte is a type of white blood cell that helps fight and prevent infection. Lymphocytes are found in blood and lymph tissue, and every organ in the body. Lymph tissue includes lymph vessels and lymph nodes. Lymphocytes normally grow in response to infection or inflammation. When they grow on their own without proper regulation, they can develop into lymphoma.

There are 3 main types of lymphocytes:

- **B lymphocytes or B cells** make antibodies. An antibody is a protein that fights infection.
- **T lymphocytes or T cells** help kill tumor cells and help control immune responses.
- **Natural killer (NK) cells** have granules (small particles) with enzymes that can kill tumor cells or cells infected with a virus.

T cell

T lymphocytes or T cells are direct fighters of foreign invaders and produce cytokines, which help activate other parts of the immune system. T cells destroy the body's own cells that have been taken over by viruses or that have become cancerous. You have normal T cells throughout your body, including in your skin.

Lymphocytes

A lymphocyte is a type of white blood cell. In primary cutaneous lymphoma, abnormal lymphocytes cause skin lesions.

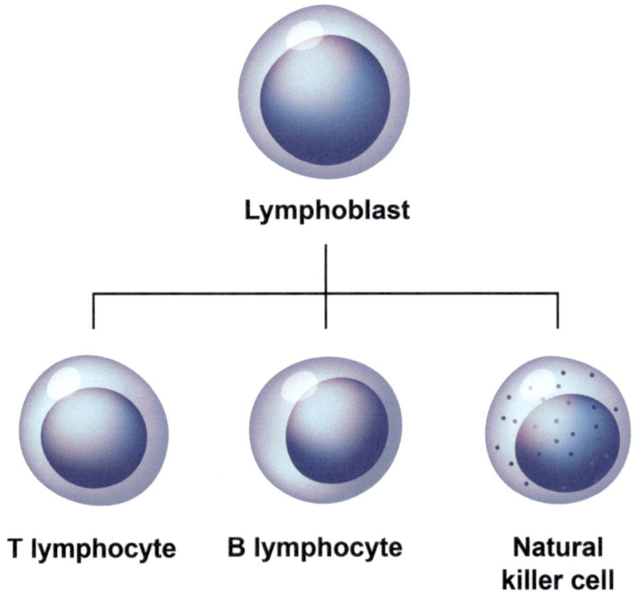

Primary cutaneous lymphomas

Primary cutaneous lymphomas (PCL) or lymphomas of the skin are a rare group of NHLs.

PCL is not a type of skin cancer. Skin cancer develops from skin cells. PCL develops from abnormal B or T lymphocytes.

There are 2 types of PCL:

- Cutaneous T-cell lymphoma (CTCL)
- Cutaneous B-cell lymphoma (CBCL)

This book will discuss treatment options for CTCL. More information on CBCL can be found at NCCN.org/patientguidelines and on the NCCN Patient Guides for Cancer app.

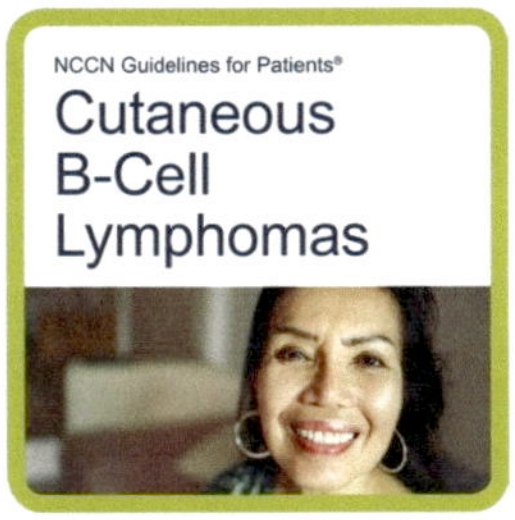

Cutaneous T-cell lymphoma

Cutaneous T-cell lymphoma (CTCL) develops when abnormal T cells grow in the skin. These abnormal cells can also grow in the blood, lymph nodes, or other areas of the body, as well as the skin. Although the skin is involved, the skin cells themselves are not cancerous.

On the skin, CTCL can cause rash-like redness, slightly raised or scaly rough patches, plaques (raised, flat-topped lesions), and sometimes skin tumors. The lesions can be itchy. Lesions may appear red, purple, or brown, and can be lighter or darker in color than the surrounding skin. It might show up as more than one type of lesion and on different parts of the skin (often in areas not exposed to the sun). Some skin lymphomas appear as a red rash over some or most of the body (known as erythroderma). Most CTCLs are slow growing (indolent) and not life threatening. However, in a small number of people, CTCL can progress to involve lymph nodes, blood, and, in rare cases, internal organs.

CTCL is treatable, but generally not curable. Most people with CTCL can live a long healthy life with ongoing care and management.

Types include:

- Mycosis fungoides (MF) and Sézary syndrome (SS) (or simply referred to as MF/SS)
- Primary cutaneous CD30+ T-cell lymphoproliferative disorders (PCTLDs)

Mycosis fungoides

Mycosis fungoides (MF) is the most common form of CTCL. It starts in the skin, but in advanced stages, MF can spread to the lymph nodes, blood, or other organs such as the spleen, liver, or lungs. MF is usually slow growing (indolent) and appears as patches, plaques, and tumors. A combination of patches, plaques, and tumors with open sores (ulceration) is possible. Symptoms include rash and itchy skin.

There are several different types of MF:

- **Folliculotropic mycosis fungoides (FMF)** affects hair follicles. Lesions are found in the head, eyebrow, or neck area and often with follicular papules and plaques. Loss of hair is common in affected sites.
- **Pagetoid reticulosis (PR) or Woringer-Kolopp disease** is characterized mostly by a single, persistent, scaly plaque, commonly involving the limbs.
- **Granulomatous slack skin (GSS)** is a rare type of CTCL where bulky, hanging skin folds are found in the armpit or groin.

Sézary syndrome

Sézary syndrome (SS) is a rare type of CTCL closely related to MF but with its own unique features. SS often causes skin redness (erythema) over most of the body called erythroderma. In SS, abnormal T cells called Sézary cells are found in the skin and blood and may cause swollen and enlarged lymph nodes (lymphadenopathy). A characteristic of Sézary cells is an abnormally shaped nucleus, described as cerebriform. On the skin, SS and MF can look alike. Blood tests are used to tell the difference. For a person to have SS, Sézary cells must be present in the blood.

Mycosis fungoides

An example of mycosis fungoides skin lesions.

Credit: CDC/ Richard S. Hibbits. https://phil.cdc.gov/Details.aspx?pid=15467

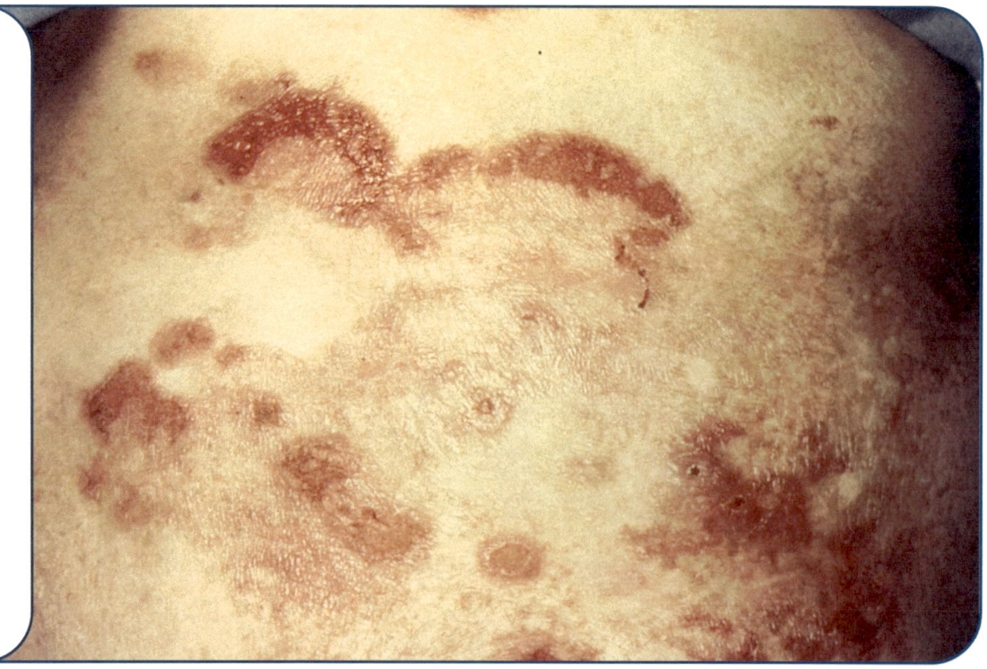

CD30+ PCTLD

Primary cutaneous CD30+ T-cell lymphoproliferative disorders (PCTLDs) are a group of diseases that include lymphomatoid papulosis (LyP), cutaneous anaplastic large cell lymphoma (ALCL), and borderline cases with overlapping features. In PCTLD, T cells or T lymphocytes that are CD30-positive (CD30+) grow and cause skin lesions or nodules. Typically, in PCTLD, more than 75 percent (75%) of T cells are CD30+. This means that at least 3 out of every 4 T cells have a protein called CD30 on their surface (CD30+).

We want your feedback!

Our goal is to provide helpful and easy-to-understand information on cancer.

Take our survey to let us know what we got right and what we could do better.

NCCN.org/patients/feedback

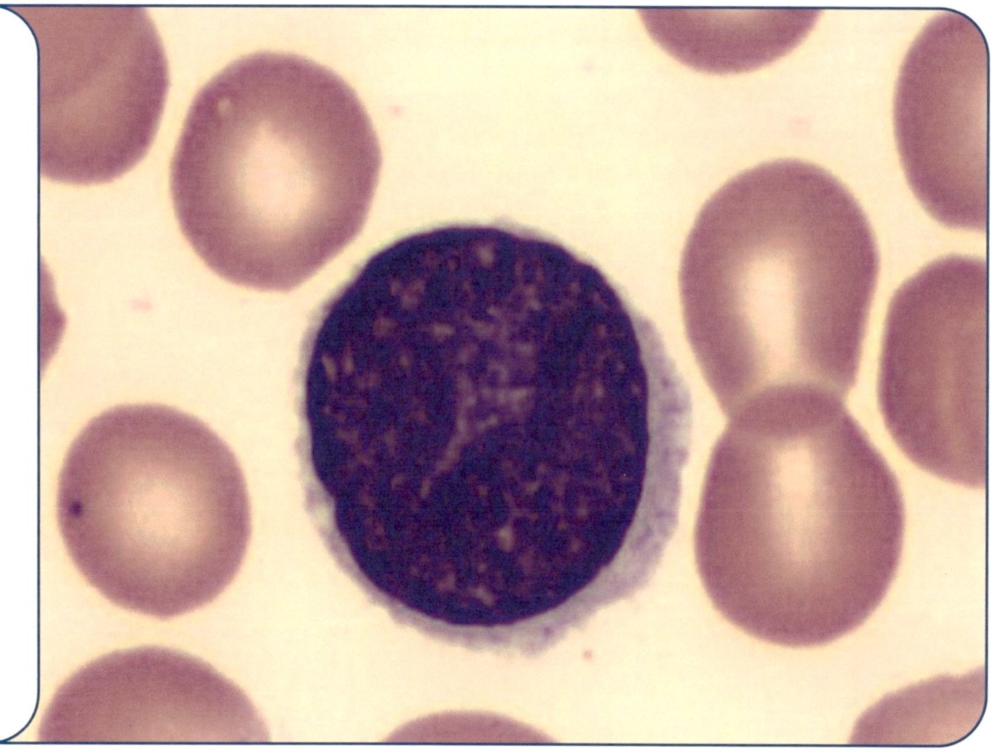

Sézary syndrome

A characteristic of Sézary cells is an abnormally shaped nucleus, described as cerebriform.

Credit: https://commons.wikimedia.org/wiki/File:Hem1SezaryCell.jpg

Key points

- Non-Hodgkin lymphoma (NHL) is a cancer that develops from lymphocytes, a type of white blood cell. Primary cutaneous lymphoma (PCL) is an NHL found in the skin. It is not skin cancer.
- Lymphocytes normally grow in response to infection or inflammation. When they grow on their own without proper regulation, they can develop into lymphoma. Lymphomas that develop on the skin are called cutaneous lymphomas.
- Cutaneous T-cell lymphoma (CTCL) develops from T-cell lymphocytes. It often appears as an itchy rash that can thicken or form a tumor.
- Mycosis fungoides (MF) is the most common form of CTCL. It starts in the skin and can spread to blood and other organs.
- In Sézary syndrome (SS), cancerous T cells called Sézary cells are found in the skin, blood, and lymph nodes.
- In primary cutaneous CD30+ T-cell lymphoproliferative disorders (PCTLDs), T cells or T lymphocytes that are CD30-positive (CD30+) grow and cause skin lesions or nodules. Types include lymphomatoid papulosis (LyP), cutaneous anaplastic large cell lymphoma (ALCL), and borderline cases with overlapping features.

Those with lymphomas of the skin should be treated at centers experienced in this type of cancer.

2

Testing for CTCL

Treatment planning starts with testing. Accurate testing is needed to diagnose and treat lymphomas of the skin such as cutaneous T-cell lymphoma (CTCL). This chapter presents an overview of possible tests you might receive and what to expect.

Test results

The diagnosis of cutaneous T-cell lymphoma (CTCL) is based mainly on a skin biopsy. Examination of the blood can detect circulating cancer cells and is part of diagnosing Sézary syndrome (SS). Results of your physical exam, blood tests, skin biopsy, and possible imaging studies will determine your treatment plan. It is important you understand what these tests mean. Ask questions about your test results. Online patient portals are one way to access your test results. Please wait to discuss the results with your doctor or health care team.

Keep these things in mind:

- It's beneficial to have a support system in place during diagnosis and treatment. Enlist the help of friends, family members, or peers who can provide transportation, meals, and emotional support. These can be different people for different tasks or change over time.
- Consider bringing someone with you to doctor visits if possible, or have someone on the phone or join you for telehealth visits.
- Don't hesitate to ask questions and take notes during appointments. Write down questions and ask a friend or family member to take notes. Caregivers should ask questions, too.
- Organize your medical documents, including insurance forms, medical records, and test results. Keep a list of contact information for your care team and update your primary care physician (PCP) regarding any changes. Include details about the specific type of cancer, treatment, and dates in your contact list.
- Set up a MyChart or health record account if it's available, which can help you track your appointments and communicate with your care team. In many places the MyChart or portal messages are not immediately seen by a nurse or physician, so ask your care team how best to communicate with them, especially in an emergency.

For possible tests and procedures, **see Guide 1.**

General health tests

Some general health tests are described next.

Medical history

A medical history is a record of all health issues and treatments you have had in your life. Be prepared to list any illness or injury and when it happened. Bring a list of old and new medicines and any over-the-counter (OTC) medicines, herbals, or supplements you take. Some supplements interact with and affect medicines that your care team may prescribe. Tell your care team about any symptoms you have. A medical history, sometimes called a health history, will help determine which treatment is best for you.

Physical exam

During a physical exam, your health care provider may:

- Check your temperature, blood pressure, pulse, and breathing rate
- Check your height and weight
- Listen to your lungs and heart
- Look in your eyes, ears, nose, and throat
- Feel and apply pressure to parts of your body to see if organs are of normal size, are soft or hard, or cause pain when touched
- Feel for enlarged lymph nodes in your neck, underarm, and groin
- Conduct a complete skin exam

Guide 1 Tests to plan treatment
Skin biopsy with pathology review and tumor/lesion testing
Medical history and physical exam, including complete skin exam
Complete blood count (CBC) with differential, comprehensive metabolic panel (CMP), and lactate dehydrogenase (LDH)
Possible: • CT with contrast of chest, abdomen, and pelvis (C/A/P) and/or PET/CT scan • Bone marrow biopsy • Lymph node biopsy • Human T-cell lymphotropic virus (HTLV) testing and other blood tests • Pregnancy test for those of childbearing age • Discussion of fertility preservation

Skin exam

A dermatologist is an expert in the skin and diseases of the skin. It is important to find a dermatologist experienced in lymphomas of the skin to conduct a skin exam. A complete skin exam looks for signs of CTCL. CTCL might appear as a rash, lumps, bumps, or tumor. A rash is an area of irritated or swollen skin. Many rashes are itchy, red, and painful.

The amount of cancer is measured using the size of your hand. One hand is equal to 1 percent (1%) of your total body surface area (BSA). In addition, any tumors will be measured by their depth, height, size, and region of the body. Keeping a photo journal might help track your skin changes over time.

You know your skin better than anyone. Tell your doctor about your normal skin color. Show the differences in where the skin looks normal and different to you. Describe any changes. Does the area itch or burn? Is it dry? Is it red or warm to the touch? Are there bumps or a raised, smooth area? Is there an odor? Share any photos.

Skin lesions

Skin is the largest organ in your body. A skin lesion is a change in color or texture in an area of the skin. Some words to describe skin lesions include patch, papule, plaque, nodule, tumor, and erythroderma.

Skin lesions

A papule is a very small, solid bump. A plaque is a raised or hardened lesion that forms on the skin, larger than a papule. Plaques sometimes become tumors on the skin.

Credit: https://commons.wikimedia.org/wiki/File:Papule_and_Plaque.svg

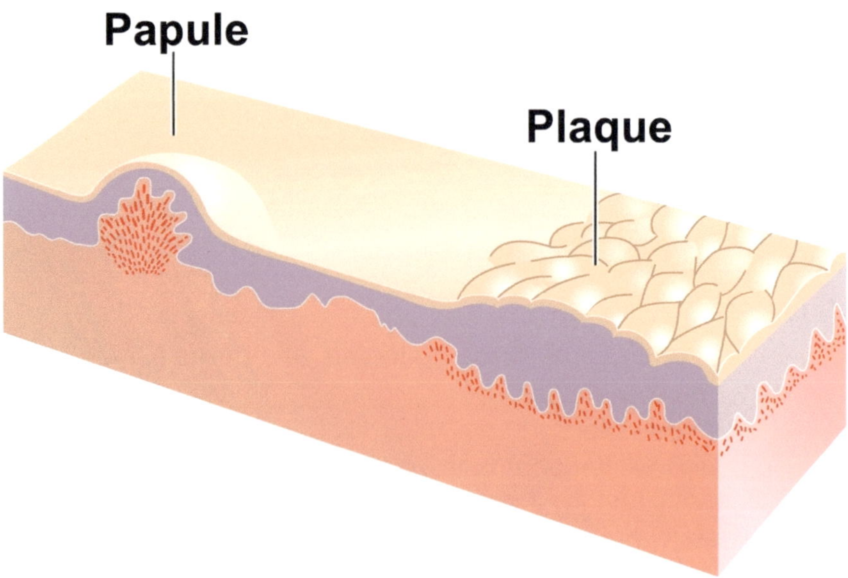

Patch

A patch is a flat, thin, pink or red lesion of any size that forms on the skin. Patches may be dry, scaly, and itchy, and may look like eczema or psoriasis. They can be lighter than surrounding skin or brown in people with darker skin. The patches may sometimes become plaques (hard, raised lesions) on the skin.

Papule

A papule is a very small, solid lump that might look like a very small pimple. Usually, papules are found in groups. Papules may be red, purple, brown, or pink.

Plaque

A plaque is a raised (elevated) or hardened (indurated) lesion of any size that forms on the skin. Plaques may be red, scaly, and itchy, and may look like eczema or psoriasis. Plaques sometimes become tumors on the skin.

Papulonodular

Papulonodular is a combination of papules and nodules found on the skin. Nodules are raised higher on the skin than papules.

Erythroderma

Erythroderma is redness of over 80% of the body's skin surface. It is an important part of recognizing and treating mycosis fungoides (MF) and Sézary syndrome (SS). Erythroderma can look like sunburn or large blotches on the skin.

Keeping a photo journal might help track skin changes over time.

Tumor

A tumor is a firm, dome-shaped mass at least 1 centimeter in size.

Ulcer

A skin ulcer is an open sore or wound on the skin.

Fertility (all genders)

Some types of treatment can impact your fertility, the ability to have children. If you think you want children in the future, ask your care team how cancer and cancer treatment might change your fertility. To preserve your fertility, you may need to take action before starting cancer treatment. Those who want to have children in the future should be referred to a fertility specialist to discuss the options before starting treatment.

Fertility preservation is all about keeping your options open, whether you know you want to have children later in life or aren't sure at the moment. Fertility and reproductive specialists can help you sort through what may be best for your situation.

More information on fertility preservation in adolescents and young adults is available at NCCN.org/patientguidelines and on the NCCN Patient Guides for Cancer app.

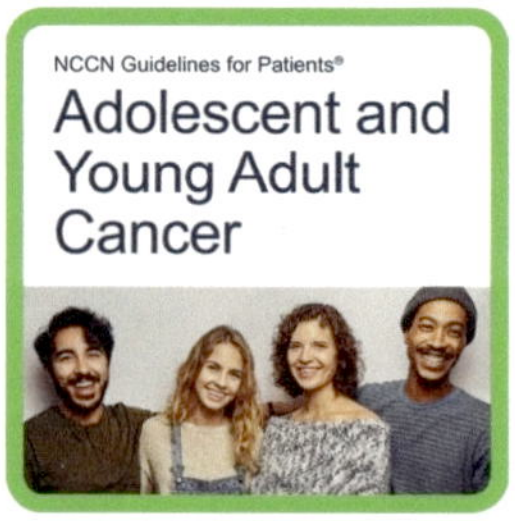

Blood tests

Blood tests check for signs of disease and how well organs are working. They require a sample of your blood, which is removed through a needle placed into a vein in your arm.

Complete blood count and differential

A complete blood count (CBC) measures the levels of red blood cells (RBCs), white blood cells (WBCs), and platelets (PLTs) in your blood. A CBC is a key test that gives a picture of your overall health. A differential counts the number of each type of WBC (neutrophils, lymphocytes, monocytes, eosinophils, and basophils). It also checks if the counts are in balance with each other.

Comprehensive metabolic panel

A comprehensive metabolic panel (CMP) measures substances in your blood. A CMP provides important information about how well your kidneys and liver are working, among other things.

HTLV

Human T-cell lymphotropic virus (HTLV) testing is used to detect an HTLV infection that could be the cause of a T-cell lymphoma. In the United States, all donated blood is screened for HTLV.

Lactate dehydrogenase

Lactate dehydrogenase (LDH) or lactic acid dehydrogenase is a protein found in most cells. Dying cells release LDH into the blood. Fast-growing cells also release LDH and cause levels of this protein to be elevated in the blood.

Pregnancy test

If planned treatment might affect pregnancy, then those who can become pregnant will be given a pregnancy test before treatment begins.

Imaging tests

Imaging tests take pictures of the inside of your body to look for cancer deposits. A radiologist, an expert in interpreting imaging tests, will write a report and send this report to your doctor. While these reports might be available to you through your patient portal or patient access system, please wait to discuss these results with your care team.

Contrast material

Contrast material is used to improve the pictures of the inside of the body. Contrast materials are substances that help enhance and improve the images of several organs and structures in the body. It is used to make the pictures clearer. The contrast is not permanent and will leave your body in your urine immediately after the test. The types of contrast vary and are different for CT and MRI.

Tell your care team if you have had allergic reactions to contrast in the past. This is important. You might be given medicines to avoid the effects of those allergies. Contrast might not be used if you have a serious allergy or if your kidneys aren't working well.

CT scan

A CT or CAT (computed tomography) scan uses x-rays and computer technology to take pictures of the inside of the body. It takes many x-rays of the same body part from different angles. All the images are combined to make one detailed picture. A CT scan of your head, neck, chest, abdomen, and pelvis may be one of the tests to look for cancer. In most cases, contrast will be used.

MRI scan

An MRI (magnetic resonance imaging) scan uses radio waves and powerful magnets to take pictures of the inside of the body. It does not use x-rays. Because of the very strong magnets used in the MRI machine, tell the technologist if you have any metal in your body. During the test, you will likely be asked to hold your breath for 10 to 20 seconds as the technician collects the images. Contrast is often used.

A closed MRI has a capsule-like design where the magnet surrounds you. An open MRI has a magnetic top and bottom, which allows for an opening on each end. Closed MRIs are more common than open MRIs, so if you have claustrophobia (a dread or fear of enclosed spaces), be sure to talk to your care team about it.

PET scan

A PET (positron emission tomography) scan uses a radioactive drug called a tracer. A tracer is a substance injected into a vein to see where cancer cells are in the body and if they are using sugar produced by your body to grow. Cancer cells show up as bright spots on PET scans. However, not all tumors will appear on a PET scan. Also, not all bright spots are cancer. It is normal for the brain, heart, kidneys, and bladder to be bright on PET. Inflammation or infection can also show up as a bright spot. When a PET scan is combined with CT, it is called a PET/CT scan.

X-ray

An x-ray is a type of radiation. In small doses, it is used to make pictures of the inside of the body. It might be referred to as a radiograph.

Biopsy

A biopsy is the removal of a sample of tissue such as skin. A biopsy is needed to diagnose CTCL. Your sample should be reviewed by a pathologist who is an expert in the diagnosis of lymphomas of the skin. The pathologist will review thin sections of the skin biopsy under a microscope. This review is often referred to as histology or histopathology review. The pathologist will note the overall appearance and the size, shape, and type of your cells.

Histology is the study of the anatomy (structure) of cells, tissues, and organs under a microscope.

A biopsy is an important part of a correct CTCL diagnosis. Diagnosing CTCL can be a challenge. It is common to have several skin biopsies in order to make a clear diagnosis.

Skin lesion biopsy

A sample of your lesion will be removed and tested to confirm a diagnosis of lymphoma of the skin. A skin lesion biopsy can be incisional or excisional. An incisional biopsy removes an area of skin using a scalpel blade. Stitches are usually required after an incisional biopsy. An excisional biopsy usually removes a larger area of skin and is done infrequently in CTCL.

Skin punch biopsy

In a skin punch biopsy, a small sample of skin and connective tissue are removed using a hand-held tool. Stitches are often used to close the opening in the skin.

Seek out support groups at your local hospital, through social media, or from those listed in the back of this book. Look to friends, relatives, neighbors, and coworkers for social support.

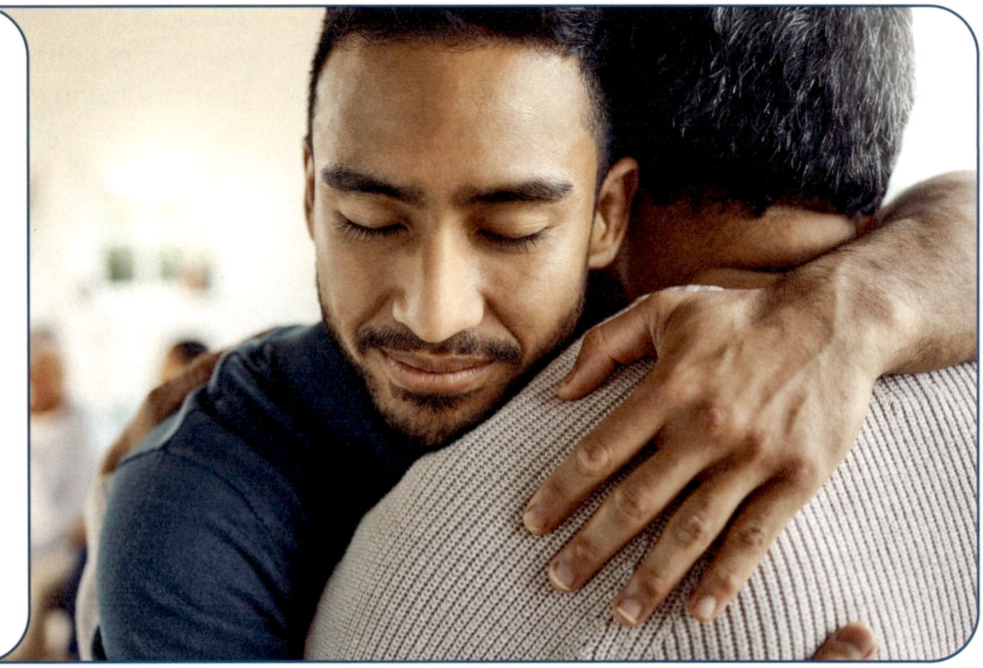

Skin shave biopsy

A skin shave biopsy removes the top layer of skin using a tool like a razor. This type of biopsy may not be recommended because it doesn't take a deep enough sample. Abnormal lymphocytes are often found under the surface of the skin.

Lymph node biopsy

Lymph nodes are usually too small to be seen or felt. Sometimes, lymph nodes can feel swollen, enlarged, hard to the touch, or don't move when pushed (fixed or immobile). A lymph node biopsy can be done using a needle biopsy procedure or as a small surgery to remove (excise) a lymph node.

Bone marrow tests

Bone marrow tests might be done in some cases.

There are 2 types of bone marrow tests that are often done at the same time:

- Bone marrow aspirate
- Bone marrow biopsy

Your bone marrow is like a sponge holding liquid and cells. An aspirate takes some of the liquid and cells out of the sponge, and a biopsy takes a piece of the sponge.

For many, this is an uncomfortable procedure. Your care team will try to make you as comfortable as possible. The samples are usually taken from the back of the hip bone (pelvis). You will likely lie on your belly or side. For an aspirate, a hollow needle will be pushed through your skin and into the bone. Liquid bone marrow will then be drawn into a syringe. For the biopsy, a wider needle will be used to remove a small piece of the bone. You may feel bone pain in your hip for a few days. Your skin may bruise.

Immunophenotyping

Immunophenotyping is a process that uses antibodies to detect the presence or absence of antigens. Antigens are proteins or markers that can be found on the surface of or inside white blood cells such as T cells. Specific groupings of antigens are normal. However, some specific patterns of antigens are found on abnormal cells.

Immunophenotyping can be done using specialized techniques called immunohistochemistry (IHC) or flow cytometry. These techniques are used to distinguish CTCL from other types of lymphoma. Immunophenotype can change as cancer progresses.

- **Mycosis fungoides (MF) and Sézary syndrome (SS)** cells are typically characterized by the following immunophenotype: CD2+, CD3+, CD5+, CD4+, CD8- (rarely CD8+ and CD4-), and they lack certain T-cell markers, such as CD7 and CD26.
- **Primary cutaneous CD30+ T-cell lymphoproliferative disorder (PCTLD) cells** are CD30-positive (CD30+).

Immunohistochemistry

Immunohistochemistry (IHC) is a special staining process that involves adding a chemical marker to immune cells. The cells are then studied using a microscope. IHC looks for the immunophenotype of cells from a skin biopsy.

CD4 and CD8 are proteins that are on two families of T lymphocytes. CD4 T cells (helper cells) help regulate functions of the immune system. CD8 T cells (killer cells) break down or rid the body of foreign substances. Most cases of CTCL come from CD4 T cells. An IHC will look for these cells and others. An IHC panel of skin biopsy may include testing for CD2, CD3, CD4, CD5, CD7, CD8, CD20, and CD30. Others might be included.

Flow cytometry

Flow cytometry is a laboratory method used to detect, identify, and count specific cells. Flow cytometry involves adding a light-sensitive dye to cells. The dyed cells are passed through a beam of light in a machine. The machine measures the number of cells, things like the size and shape of the cells, and other unique features of the cells. Flow cytometry may be used on cells from circulating (peripheral) blood, bone marrow, or a biopsy. The most common use of flow cytometry is in the identification of markers on cells, particularly in the immune system (called immunophenotyping). In CTCL, flow cytometry is often used to count the number of Sézary cells or CTCL cells in the blood.

Testing for CTCL biomarker and genetic changes

Biomarker and genetic tests are used to learn more about your type of CTCL, to guide treatment, and to determine the likely path your cancer will take (prognosis). This genetic testing is different from family history genetic testing or genetic cancer risk testing. This testing looks for changes only in the CTCL cells that have developed over time, and not changes in the rest of your body's cells.

Inside our cells are DNA molecules. These molecules are tightly packaged into what is called a chromosome. Chromosomes contain most of the genetic information in a cell. Normal human cells contain 23 pairs of chromosomes for a total of 46 chromosomes. Each chromosome contains thousands of genes. Genes are coded instructions for the proteins your cells make. A mutation is when something goes wrong in the genetic code. Proteins are written like this: CD4. Genes are written with italics like this: *TCR.* When a gene or protein is found (expressed), it is shown with a plus sign (+) like this: CD4+. When a gene or protein has not been found, it is written with a negative sign (-) like this CD4-.

CTCL mutation testing

A sample of your skin, lymph node, blood, or bone marrow might be used to see if the cancer cells have any specific mutations. Some mutations can be targeted with specific therapies. This is separate from the genetic testing for mutations that you may have inherited from your biological parents.

CTCL cells can have changes in genes and chromosomes. Some mutations may determine the type of treatment given. Subtle new drug-resistant mutations may occur over time. Mutations can also happen during treatment. Mutation testing is used to look for these new mutations. Some mutations lead to resistance to certain targeted therapies. There are many possible mutations. Ask your care team for more information.

FISH

Fluorescence in situ hybridization (FISH) is a method that involves special dyes called probes that attach to pieces of DNA. Since this test doesn't need growing cells, it can be performed on a blood sample.

FISH can find translocations that are too small to be seen with other methods. A translocation occurs when parts of two chromosomes switch with one another. However, FISH can only be used for known changes. It cannot detect all the possible changes found within the chromosomes or genes. For example, FISH is used to detect *TP63* gene rearrangements by attaching probes to *TP63* (3q28) and *TBL1XR1/TP63*.

Gene rearrangements

Normal T cells break their DNA in certain ways to create diversity within your immune system. In a tumor, all cancer cells are derived from the same original cell. In CTCL that cell is a T cell. When that one T cell divides many times, the entire group of T cells is called clonal or the tumor is described as having clonality. Clonal T cells should have the same T-cell receptor and the same T-cell receptor gene sequence. Pathologists have tests to determine if a group of cells is clonal or not. This is commonly described as TCR.

Biomarker and genetic testing is used to detect T-cell rearrangements commonly found in CTCL. This information can be helpful when diagnosing and treating CTCL. SS has a clonal rearrangement of *TCR* in the blood.

Key points

- Tests check for signs of disease, determine how well organs are working, and assess treatment results.
- Skin lesions can appear anywhere on the body. Lesions may look like papules, patches, plaques, or nodules.
- A biopsy is needed to diagnose lymphomas of the skin such as cutaneous T-cell lymphomas (CTCLs). Your biopsy should be reviewed by a pathologist who is an expert in the diagnosis of CTCL.
- A sample from your biopsy may undergo lab tests to learn more about your lymphoma and help you and your care team choose the best treatment for you.

3

MF and SS cancer staging

A cancer stage is a way to describe how much cancer is in your body and where it is located. It is used to make treatment decisions. Cancer staging for mycosis fungoides (MF)/Sézary syndrome (SS) is different than for other lymphomas of the skin. Although the same staging system is used, MF and SS are treated differently.

TNMB scores

The tumor, node, metastasis (TNM) system is used to stage many cancers. In this system, the letters T, N, and M describe different areas of cancer growth. Based on biopsy and other test results, each letter will be assigned a score or number. The higher the number, the larger the tumor or the more the cancer has spread to lymph nodes or other organs. These scores will be combined to assign the cancer a stage. A TNM example might look like this: T1N0M0 or T1, N0, M0.

Staging in MF/SS looks slightly different than in other cancers. It is referred to as TNMB or tumor, node, metastasis, blood.

- **T is for skin** – In mycosis fungoides/Sézary syndrome (MF/SS), tumor refers to type and number of tumors covering the skin. Staging looks for the presence of tumors, patches, papules, plaques, or reddening of the skin (erythema) and how much body surface area (BSA) is affected.
- **N is for node** – This refers to if abnormal T lymphocytes are found in lymph nodes.
- **M is for metastasis** – In MF/SS, metastasis refers to if cancer is found in internal (visceral) organs or bone marrow.
- **B is for blood** – This refers to if abnormal T lymphocytes are found in circulating (peripheral) blood.

T = Skin

In MF/SS, the amount of cancer is measured by evaluating what percent of your skin is affected by lymphoma. One hand is equal to 1 percent (1%) of your total body surface area (BSA). In addition, any tumors will be measured by their depth, height, size, and region of the body. Tumors are often measured in centimeters (cm).

- **T1** – Patches, papules, and/or plaques cover less than 10% BSA
- **T2** – Patches, papules, and/or plaques cover 10% or more BSA
  - **T2a** is patch only
  - **T2b** is plaque with or without patch
- **T3** – One or more tumors of 1 cm or more in size
- **T4** – Reddening, thickening, or involvement of the skin (erythema) covering 80% or more BSA

N = Node

There are hundreds of lymph nodes throughout your body. Lymph nodes work as filters to help fight infection and remove harmful things. They also produce lymphocytes. As abnormal T lymphocytes multiply, they can distort or overtake the lymph node.

Abnormal lymph nodes are any that can be felt on physical exam as firm, irregular, clustered, fixed, or 1.5 cm or more in diameter. Node groups examined on physical exam include neck (cervical), above the collarbone (supraclavicular), arm (epitrochlear), armpit (axillary), and groin (inguinal).

- **N0** means that there are no abnormal T lymphocytes found in lymph nodes.
- **N1** means that there are some abnormal T lymphocytes found in lymph nodes.
- **N2** means that there are many abnormal T lymphocytes or clusters found in lymph nodes.
- **N3** means that abnormal T lymphocytes have altered the structure of lymph nodes. This is called lymph node (nodal) disease.

M = Metastasis

Cancer that has spread to distant parts of the body is usually called metastatic. It is shown as M1. In MF/SS, cancer can spread to bone marrow or visceral (internal, solid) organs such as the spleen, liver, or lungs.

- **M0** means no cancer is found in the bone marrow or internal organs.
- **M1A** means cancer is found in bone marrow.
- **M1B** means cancer is found in visceral organs.

B = Blood

Peripheral blood circulates throughout your body (bloodstream). The amount of abnormal T cells found in the blood will be measured.

- **B0 (no or very low blood involvement)** – No blood involvement or very small amounts (less than 5% or 250 cells/mm^3) of CD4+/CD26- or CD4+/CD7- Sézary cells are found in the blood.
- **B1 (low blood tumor burden)** – More than 5% but less than 1000/µL of peripheral (circulating) blood lymphocytes are Sézary cells.
- **B2 (high blood tumor burden)** – More than 1000/µL Sézary cells are found. A diagnosis of SS requires B2 involvement.

MF/SS numbered stages

Number stages range from stage 1 to stage 4, with 4 being the most advanced. These stages are written as stage I, stage II, stage III, and stage IV. Not all cancers are described this way. Stages are defined by TNMB scores.

For MF/SS numbered cancer stages, **see Guide 2.**

Guide 2
MF/SS cancer stages

Stage 1	Stage 1A Limited skin involvement	• T1, N0, M0, B0 or B1
	Stage 1B Skin only disease	• T2, N0, M0, B0 or B1
Stage 2	Stage 2A	• T1 or T2, N1 or N2, M0, B0 or B1
	Stage 2B Tumor stage disease	• T3, N0 or N1 or N2, M0, B0 or B1
Stage 3	Stage 3A Erythrodermic disease	• T4, N0 or N1 or N2, M0, B0
	Stage 3B Erythrodermic disease	• T4, N0 or N1 or N2, M0, B1
Stage 4	Stage $4A_1$ Sézary syndrome	• Any T, N0 or N1 or N2, M0, B2
	Stage $4A_2$ Can be SS or MF	• Any T, N3, M0, Any B
	Stage 4B Visceral disease (SS or MF)	• Any T, Any N, M1A or M1B, Any B

Stage 1A – Limited skin involvement

Limited patches, papules, and/or plaques cover less than 10% of the skin (T1). Cancer is not found in lymph nodes (N0) or visceral organs (M0).

Stage 1B – Skin only disease

Stage 1B has more skin involvement than stage 1A. Patches, papules, and/or plaques cover 10% or more of the skin (T2). Cancer is not found in lymph nodes (N0) or visceral organs (M0).

Stage 2A

Any amount of the skin surface is covered with patches or plaques (T1 or T2). Cancer is found in the lymph nodes (N1 or N2).

Stage 2B – Tumor stage disease

One or more tumors 1 cm or more in size are found on the skin (T3). Cancer may (N1 or N2) or may not (N0) be in the lymph nodes. It may (B1) or may not (B0) be found in blood.

Stage 3A – Erythrodermic disease

In erythrodermic disease, nearly all of the skin (more than 80%) is reddened (erythema) (T4), but little disease is found inside the body. Patches, plaques, or tumors may be found on the skin. Cancer may (N1 or N2) or may not (N0) be in the lymph nodes. There is no visceral (M0) or blood (B0) involvement.

Stage 3B – Erythrodermic disease

This is the same as 3A, except that a small amount of cancer is found in the blood (B1).

Stage $4A_1$ – Sézary syndrome

Stage 4A1 has significant disease in the blood, including a high number of Sézary cells (B2). Skin can be any stage (any T). Cancer may (N1 or N2) or may not (N0) be in the lymph nodes.

Stage $4A_2$ – SS or MF

Stage 4A2 has significant disease in the lymph nodes. Skin can be any stage (any T). Abnormal T lymphocytes have altered the structure of the lymph node (N3). Cancer may be found in blood. A diagnosis of SS requires B2 blood involvement.

Stage 4B – Visceral disease (SS or MF)

Stage 4B has more significant disease in the organs. Skin can be any stage (any T). Lymph nodes can be any stage (any N). Cancer has spread to bone marrow (M1A) or internal (visceral) organs (M1B). There may be blood involvement (any B). MF or SS can be stage 4B.

Key points

- A cancer stage is a way to describe how much cancer is in your body and where it is located. It is used to make treatment decisions.
- Staging for mycosis fungoides (MF)/ Sézary syndrome (SS) looks slightly different than for other cancers. It is referred to as TNMB or tumor, node, metastasis (visceral), blood.
- Staging may change as cancer progresses.
- MF can be stage 1, 2, 3, $4A_2$, or 4B.
- In SS, cancerous T cells called Sézary cells are found in the skin, lymph nodes, and blood. SS can be stage $4A_1$, $4A_2$, or 4B.

Those with lymphomas of the skin should be treated at centers experienced in this type of cancer.

4

Treating CTCL

This chapter presents an overview of the possible types of treatment and what to expect. Not everyone will receive the same treatment. Treatment options are based on many factors. Together, you and your care team will choose a treatment plan that is best for you.

Care team

CTCL is treatable, but generally not curable. You can live a long healthy life with ongoing care and management.

Treating cancer takes a team approach. Treatment decisions should involve a multidisciplinary team (MDT). An MDT is a team of health care and psychosocial care professionals from different professional backgrounds who have knowledge (expertise) and experience in your type of cancer. This team is united in the planning and implementing of your treatment. Ask who will coordinate your care.

Some members of your care team will be with you throughout cancer treatment, while others will only be there for parts of it. Get to know your care team and help them get to know you.

Depending on your diagnosis, your team might include the following specialists:

- **A dermatologist** specializes in the diagnosis and treatment of skin diseases.
- **A hematologist or hematologic oncologist** is a medical expert in blood diseases and blood cancers. Other types of oncologists include medical, radiation, and surgical oncologists.
- **A pathologist, dermatopathologist, or hematopathologist** analyzes the cells and tissues removed during a biopsy and provides cancer diagnosis, staging, and information about biomarker testing.
- **A radiation oncologist** treats cancer using radiation therapy (RT).
- **Oncology nurses** provide your hands-on care, like giving systemic therapy, managing your care, answering questions, and helping you cope with side effects.
- **An advanced practice nurse (APN) or a physician assistant (PA)** help provide an extra layer of support with your cancer-related symptoms.
- **Oncology pharmacists** are experts in knowing how to use medicines to treat cancer and to manage symptoms and side effects.
- **Palliative care specialists** concentrate on preventing and alleviating suffering and improving quality of life.
- **An occupational therapist** helps people with the tasks of daily living.
- **A physical therapist** helps people move with greater comfort and ease.

- **Psychologists and psychiatrists** are mental health experts who can help manage issues such as depression, anxiety, or other mental health conditions that can affect how you think and feel.
- **Social workers** help people solve and cope with problems in their everyday lives. Clinical social workers also diagnose and treat mental, behavioral, and emotional issues. The anxiety a person feels when diagnosed with cancer might be managed by a social worker in some cancer centers. They, or other designated professionals, can help navigate the complexities of financial and insurance stresses.
- **Spiritual care specialists** identify and support those with spiritual distress or unmet spiritual needs.
- **A research team** helps to collect research data and coordinate care if you are in a clinical trial. Clinical trials help bring new therapies to patients and advance the treatment for everyone. Consider asking your care team about access to clinical trials.

You know your body better than anyone

Help your care team understand:

- ✓ How you feel
- ✓ What you need
- ✓ What is working and what is not

Keep a list of names and contact information for each member of your team. This will make it easier for you and anyone involved in your care to know whom to contact with questions or concerns.

Get to know your care team and help them get to know you.

Preventing pregnancy during treatment

Cancer and cancer treatment can affect the ovaries and damage sperm. If you become pregnant during chemotherapy, radiation therapy, or other types of systemic therapy, serious birth defects can occur. Speak with your care team about preventing pregnancy while being treated for cancer. Hormonal birth control may or may not be recommended, so ask your doctor about options such as intrauterine devices (IUDs) and barrier methods. Types of barrier methods include condoms, diaphragms, cervical caps, and the contraceptive sponge.

Those with ovaries

Those who can become pregnant will have a pregnancy test before starting treatment. Cancer treatment can hurt the developing baby if you are or become pregnant during treatment. Therefore, birth control to prevent pregnancy during and after treatment is recommended. If you are pregnant or breastfeeding at the time of your cancer diagnosis, certain treatments will need to be avoided.

Menstruation, menses, menstrual flow, or your period may stop during treatment, but often returns within 2 years after treatment in those 35 years of age and under. It is still possible to become pregnant even though you might not have a period. Therefore, birth control is recommended during and after treatment. Consult your doctor for the best time to plan a pregnancy.

Those with testicles

Cancer and cancer treatment can damage sperm. Therefore, use contraception (birth control) such as condoms to prevent pregnancy during and immediately after cancer treatment.

Standard of care is the best-known way to treat a particular disease based on past clinical trials. There may be more than one treatment regimen that is considered standard of care. Ask your care team what treatment options are available and if a clinical trial might be right for you.

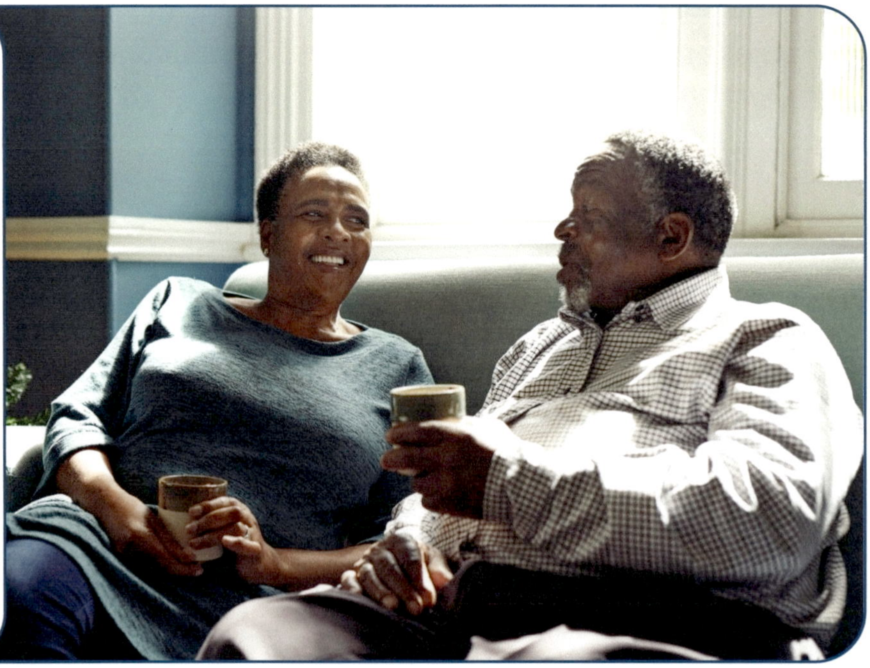

Skin-directed therapy

Types of therapy focused on the skin include topical therapy, local radiation, and phototherapy.

Topical therapy

A topical treatment is put on the surface of the skin. It might be a lotion (cream), gel, or ointment. Types of topical therapy are described next.

- **Corticosteroids (steroids)** are used to reduce inflammation. Steroids can be topical or intralesional. An intralesional steroid is injected directly into a lesion on or just below the skin.
- **Imiquimod** is used to treat certain types of flat, scaly growths on the skin. Brand names include Aldara and Zyclara.
- **Nitrogen mustard (mechlorethamine hydrochloride)** stops or slows the growth of cancer. Brand names include Valchlor and Ledaga.
- **Retinoids** are products related to vitamin A. Examples include bexarotene (Targretin gel) and tazarotene (Tazorac Gel, Tazorac Cream).
- **Carmustine** is a chemotherapy that stops or slows the growth of cancer. Topical carmustine (BiCNU) is applied to lesions.

Local radiation therapy

Local radiation therapy (RT) treats the skin lesion. Involved-site radiation therapy (ISRT) is a type of local radiation. It can be used on lymph nodes and/or skin lesions. The type of radiation is usually electrons. Some with CTCL may see a benefit with low doses of radiation.

Phototherapy

Phototherapy uses different ultraviolet (UV) light wavelengths to treat skin lesions or tumors.

Types include:

- **Ultraviolet B (UVB)** – exposes the skin to an artificial UVB light source for a set length of time on a regular schedule.
- **Narrowband ultraviolet B (NB-UVB)** – uses a very specific UV wavelength.
- **Photochemotherapy or psoralen plus ultraviolet A (PUVA)** – combines psoralen (P) with UVA. Psoralen is a type of medicine taken by mouth (orally) that causes your skin to be sensitive to light. After taking psoralen, the skin is exposed to long-wave UV light.
- **Ultraviolet A1 (UVA1)** – penetrates deep into the skin causing T cells to die.

Often, UVB or NB-UVB is used for patch or thin plaques and PUVA or UVA1 is used for thicker plaques or tumors.

UV can increase your risk of some skin cancers. Phototherapy may not be favored in those with a history of skin cancer, or who have had melanoma.

Radiation therapy

Radiation therapy (RT) uses high-energy radiation from x-rays, photons, electrons, and other sources to kill cancer cells and shrink tumors. RT can be given alone or with other treatments. Treatment may focus on individual tumors, a small area/region of the body, the entire surface of the skin, or specific lymph nodes. RT may be used as supportive care or palliative care to help ease pain or discomfort caused by cancer. RT in CTCL often involves use of electrons which only affects tissues a couple millimeters deep.

EBRT

External beam radiation therapy (EBRT) uses a machine outside of the body to aim radiation at the tumor(s) or areas of the body.

The most common types of EBRT that may be used to treat CTCL include:

- **Involved-site radiation therapy (ISRT)** targets a specific area of skin. It can also be used to treat specific lymph nodes with cancer.
- **Total skin electron beam therapy (TSEBT)** treats the entire skin surface. You might stand on a rotating platform to receive this treatment.

Warnings about supplements and drug interactions

You might be asked to stop taking or avoid certain herbal supplements when on a systemic therapy. Some supplements can affect the ability of a drug to do its job. This is called a drug interaction.

It is critical to speak with your care team about any supplements you may be taking. Some examples include:

- Turmeric
- Ginkgo biloba
- Green tea extract
- St. John's Wort
- Antioxidants

Certain medicines can also affect the ability of a drug to do its job. Antacids, heart or blood pressure medicine, and antidepressants are just some of the medicines that might interact with a systemic therapy or supportive care medicines given during systemic therapy. Therefore, it is very important to tell your care team about any medicines, vitamins, over-the-counter (OTC) drugs, herbals, or supplements you are taking.

Bring a list with you to every visit.

Systemic therapy

Systemic therapy works throughout the body. It includes retinoids, chemotherapy, targeted therapy, and immunotherapy. Systemic therapy might be used alone or with other therapies.

Extracorporeal photopheresis

Photopheresis, also known as extracorporeal photopheresis (ECP), is a medical treatment that removes blood from the body using a machine. The machine separates out the white blood cells. These white cells are exposed to a medicine called 8-methoxypsoralen (8-MOP) followed by ultraviolet A (UVA) radiation. Then the blood with the treated white blood cells is returned to your body.

Chemotherapy

Chemotherapy kills fast-growing cells throughout the body, including cancer cells and normal cells. There are many chemotherapies used to treat primary cutaneous lymphomas.

Retinoids

Retinoids are products related to vitamin A that can stop the growth of cancer cells. When taken by mouth (orally), they work throughout the body.

The goal of treatment is to improve your condition and to maintain this improvement for as long as possible.

Targeted therapy

Targeted therapy focuses on specific or unique features of cancer cells. Targeted therapies seek out how cancer cells grow, divide, and move in the body. These drugs stop the action of molecules that help cancer cells grow and/or survive.

Immunotherapy

Immunotherapy is a drug therapy that increases the activity of your immune system. By doing so, it improves your body's ability to find and destroy cancer cells. Immunotherapy can be given alone or with other types of treatment.

Clinical trials

A clinical trial is a type of medical research study. After being developed and tested in a laboratory, potential new ways of treating cancer need to be studied in people. If found to be safe and effective in a clinical trial, a drug, device, or treatment approach may be approved by the U.S. Food and Drug Administration (FDA).

Everyone with cancer should carefully consider all of the treatment options available for their cancer type, including standard treatments and clinical trials. Talk to your doctor about whether a clinical trial may make sense for you.

Phases

Most cancer clinical trials focus on treatment. Treatment trials are done in phases.

- **Phase 1 trials** study the dose, safety, and side effects of an investigational drug or treatment approach. They also look for early signs that the drug or approach is helpful.
- **Phase 2 trials** study how well the drug or approach works against a specific type of cancer.
- **Phase 3 trials** test the drug or approach against a standard treatment. If the results are good, it may be approved by the FDA.
- **Phase 4 trials** study the long-term safety and benefit of an FDA-approved treatment.

Finding a clinical trial

In the United States

NCCN Cancer Centers
NCCN.org/cancercenters

The National Cancer Institute (NCI)
cancer.gov/about-cancer/treatment/clinical-trials/search

Worldwide

The U.S. National Library of Medicine (NLM)
clinicaltrials.gov

Need help finding a clinical trial?

NCI's Cancer Information Service (CIS)
1.800.4.CANCER (1.800.422.6237)
cancer.gov/contact

Who can enroll?

Every clinical trial has rules for joining, called eligibility criteria. The rules may be about age, cancer type and stage, treatment history, lab tests, or general health. These requirements ensure that participants are alike in specific ways and that the trial is as safe as possible for the participants.

Informed consent

Clinical trials are managed by a group of experts called a research team. The research team will review the study with you in detail, including its purpose and the risks and benefits of joining. All of this information is also provided in an informed consent form. Read the form carefully and ask questions before signing it. Take time to discuss with family, friends, or others whom you trust. Keep in mind that you can leave and seek treatment outside of the clinical trial at any time.

Start the conversation

Don't wait for your doctor to bring up clinical trials. Start the conversation and learn about all of your treatment options. If you find a study that you may be eligible for, ask your treatment team if you meet the requirements. If you have already started standard treatment you may not be eligible for certain clinical trials. Try not to be discouraged if you cannot join. New clinical trials are always becoming available.

Frequently asked questions

There are many myths and misconceptions surrounding clinical trials. The possible benefits and risks are not well understood by many with cancer.

Will I get a placebo?
Placebos (inactive versions of real medicines) are almost never used alone in cancer clinical trials. It is common to receive either a placebo with a standard treatment, or a new drug with a standard treatment. You will be informed, verbally and in writing, if a placebo is part of a clinical trial before you enroll.

Do I have to pay to be in a clinical trial?
It depends on the study, your health insurance, and the state in which you live. In general, procedures, drugs, or tests that are considered standard of care will be billed to you or your insurance, whereas those considered research are covered by the trial sponsor. Your treatment team and the research team can help determine if you are responsible for any costs.

Hematopoietic cell transplant

A hematopoietic stem cell is an immature cell that can develop into any type of blood cell. A hematopoietic cell transplant (HCT) replaces hematopoietic stem cells that have been destroyed by high doses of chemotherapy and/or radiation therapy as part of the transplant process. You might hear it called a stem cell transplant (SCT) or a bone marrow transplant (BMT). This book will refer to it as HCT. HCTs are performed in specialized centers.

There are 2 types of HCT:

- **Autologous** – stem cells come from you
- **Allogeneic** – stem cells come from a donor who may or may not be related to you

In some cases, an allogeneic HCT is a treatment option. It is used to cure MF/SS. The steps of an allogeneic HCT are described next.

Allogeneic transplant

An allogeneic hematopoietic cell transplant (allogeneic HCT) uses healthy stem cells from a donor. The donor may or may not be related to you. Before an HCT, treatment is needed to destroy bone marrow cells. This is called conditioning and it creates room for the healthy donor stem cells and eliminates any remaining lymphoma cells. Your blood will be in a weakened state after conditioning until the donor stem cells settle in and take over as your new blood supply. Conditioning also weakens the immune system so your body won't kill the transplanted cells. Chemotherapy and/or radiation is used for conditioning.

After conditioning, you will receive a transfusion of the healthy stem cells from a donor matched to you. A transfusion is a slow injection of blood products into a vein. This can take several hours. The transplanted stem cells will travel to your bone marrow and grow. New, healthy blood cells will form. This is called engraftment. It usually takes about 2 to 4 weeks. Until then, you will have little or no immune defense. You may need to stay in a very clean room at the hospital or be given antibiotics to prevent or treat infection. Transfusions are also possible. A red blood cell transfusion is used to prevent bleeding and to treat anemia (below normal red blood cell count). A platelet transfusion is used to treat a low platelet count or bleeding. While waiting for the cells to engraft, you will likely feel tired and weak.

The goal of the transplant is for the new immune system to recognize what remains of the CTCL as foreign and destroy it and to provide you with new, healthy bone marrow.

Possible side effects

Every treatment has side effects. You will be monitored for infections, decreases in your blood counts that require blood transfusions, disease relapse, and graft-versus-host disease (GVHD). In GVHD, the donor cells attack your normal, healthy tissue. There are treatments for GVHD. Ask your care team about the possible side effects or complications of HCT and how this might affect your quality of life.

More information on GVHD can be found at NCCN.org/patientguidelines and on the NCCN Patient Guides for Cancer app.

General supportive care

Supportive care will be specific to your needs. Supportive care is health care given to prevent, reduce, and relieve suffering, and to improve quality of life. Supportive care might include pain relief, palliative care, emotional or spiritual support, financial aid, or family counseling. Tell your care team how you are feeling and about any side effects so they can be managed. Supportive care, best supportive care, and palliative care often mean the same thing.

It is very important to take care of yourself by eating well, drinking plenty of fluids, exercising, and doing things that make you feel energized.

Side effects

All cancer treatments can cause unwanted health issues called side effects. Side effects depend on many factors. These factors include the drug type and dose, length of treatment, and the person. Some side effects may be harmful to your health. Others may just be unpleasant. Treatment can cause several side effects. Some are very serious.

Ask for a complete list of side effects of your treatments. Also, tell your treatment team about any new or worsening symptoms. There may be ways to help you feel better. There are also ways to prevent some side effects. You will be monitored closely for side effects.

Late effects

Late effects are side effects that occur months or years after a disease is diagnosed or after treatment has ended. Late effects may be caused by cancer or cancer treatment. They may include physical, mental, and social health issues, and second cancers. The sooner late effects are treated the better. Ask your care team about what late effects could occur. This will help you know what to look for.

Survivorship

A person is a cancer survivor from the time of diagnosis until the end of life. After treatment, your health will be monitored for side effects of treatment and the return of cancer. This is part of your survivorship care plan. It is important to keep any follow-up doctor visits and imaging test appointments. Seek good routine medical care, including regular doctor visits for preventive care and cancer screening.

A personalized survivorship care plan will contain a summary of possible long-term effects of treatment called late effects and list follow-up tests. Find out how your primary care provider will coordinate with specialists for your follow-up care.

Key points

- CTCL is treatable, but generally not curable. You can live a long healthy life with ongoing care and management.
- Skin-directed therapy focuses on the skin and includes topical therapy, local radiation, and phototherapy.
- Systemic therapy works throughout the body. It includes chemotherapy, targeted therapy, immunotherapy, extracorporeal photopheresis (ECP), and retinoids.
- Radiation therapy (RT) uses high-energy radiation from x-rays, electrons, photons, and other sources to kill cancer cells and shrink tumors.
- Clinical trials study how safe and helpful tests and cancer treatments are for people.
- Supportive care is health care that relieves symptoms caused by cancer or its treatment and improves quality of life.
- All cancer treatments can cause unwanted health issues called side effects. You will be monitored for side effects, infection, and other treatment-related issues.

All cancer treatments can cause unwanted health issues called side effects. It is important to tell your care team about all of your side effects so they can be managed.

5

Mycosis fungoides

Mycosis fungoides is a chronic disease that starts in the skin, but in advanced stages can spread to the lymph nodes, blood, or other organs. Depending on the cancer stage, treatment might be a skin-directed therapy or a combination of systemic therapy with skin-directed therapy. The goal of treatment is to improve your condition and to maintain this improvement for as long as possible. Together, you and your care team will choose a treatment plan that is best for you.

The goal of treatment is to improve your condition and to maintain this improvement for as long as possible. Treatment will be based on the cancer stage, if any and what treatments were given before, and other factors. If cancer in the blood (B1 involvement) is suspected, then treatment may follow stage 3 (erythrodermic disease).

Stage 1A

In stage 1A, cancer is limited to a small area on the skin (T1). The amount of cancer is measured by evaluating what percent of your skin is affected by lymphoma. One hand is equal to 1 percent (1%) of your total body surface area (BSA). In stage 1A, less than 10% of the skin (BSA) is covered in patches, papules, and/or plaques.

Primary treatment

Primary treatment is the first treatment given. Treatment options focus on skin-directed therapies. These therapies may be used alone or with other skin-directed therapies or with systemic (drug) therapy. Preferred systemic therapy options include bexarotene (Targretin), interferon, or methotrexate.

- A complete response (CR) is described as remission or a disease-free period. In order to maintain remission for as long as possible, maintenance therapy is often given. Maintenance therapy uses the same treatment, but often at a lower dose.
- In a partial response (PR), treatment is working, but cancer remains. You will likely continue the same treatment until a CR.

Relapse

When cancer returns after a disease-free period, it is called a relapse. Relapse can happen after a CR or PR. Treatment is based on cancer stage.

Progression

Disease progression is cancer that is growing or spreading. If cancer progresses higher than stage 1A, then treatment is based on the new stage.

Persistent

T1 skin disease that persists, but has not progressed, may be treated with a different skin-directed therapy. Treatment aims to reduce the amount of cancer before starting treatment for refractory disease.

Refractory

When cancer appears resistant to multiple therapies, it is called refractory. Treatment might be systemic therapy with or without skin-directed therapies as found in stage 1B and 2A, radiation therapy if not used before, or a clinical trial.

Stage 1B and 2A

In stage 1B, patches, papules, and/or plaques cover 10% or more of the skin (T2). Cancer is not found in lymph nodes (N0) or visceral organs (M0).

In stage 2A, any amount of the skin surface is covered with patches or plaques (T1 or T2). There is some involvement of lymph nodes, but not enough to alter the structure of lymph nodes (N1 or N2). If cancer is found in the blood (B1), it might be treated as stage 3 erythrodermic disease.

Treatment for stage 1B and 2A is based on the amount of skin disease called burden. The lower the amount of skin disease, the lower the skin disease burden.

Mycosis fungoides

An example of mycosis fungoides skin lesions found on the arm.

Credit: https://commons.wikimedia.org/wiki/File:Mycosis_fungoide.JPG

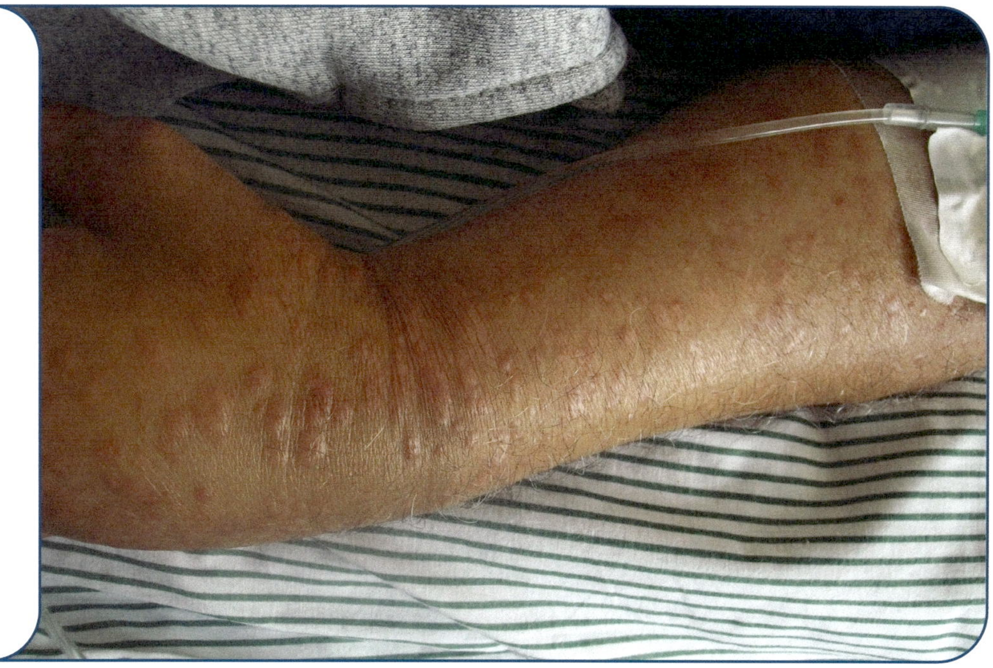

Lower skin disease burden

Lower skin disease burden is mostly patch disease. A limited area of the skin is involved. Treatment focuses on limited or local skin-directed therapies. These therapies might be used alone or in combination with other skin-directed therapies or with systemic therapy. For systemic therapy options, **see Guide 3.**

Higher skin disease burden

Higher skin disease burden is mostly plaque disease. The goal of treatment is to improve your condition and to reduce the amount of cancer burden.

Treatment options include:

- Skin-directed therapies for general skin involvement
- Systemic therapy alone or with skin-directed therapies. For systemic therapy options, **see Guide 3.**

Relapse

When cancer returns after a disease-free period, it is called a relapse. Treatment will be based on the cancer stage, what treatments were given before, and other factors.

Progression

If cancer progresses to higher than stage 1B or 2A, then the cancer will be restaged. Treatment will be based on the new stage.

Persistent

Persistent disease is disease that remains after completing primary treatment. Treatment aims to reduce the amount of cancer before choosing a treatment for refractory disease.

Guide 3 Preferred systemic therapies: Stage 1B and 2A
Bexarotene (Targretin)
Brentuximab vedotin (Adcetris)
Interferon
Methotrexate
Mogamulizumab (Poteligeo)
Romidepsin (Istodax)
Vorinostat (Zolinza)

Refractory

When cancer appears resistant to multiple therapies, it is called refractory.

Treatment options include:

- Clinical trial
- Total skin electron beam therapy (TSEBT), if not used before
- Treatments found under Stage 2B below

Stage 2B

Stage 2B is also called tumor stage disease. In this stage, one or more tumors 1 cm or larger in size are found on the skin. Treatment is based on if the tumors are limited or widespread. Abnormal T cells may be found in the lymph nodes and/or blood.

Limited tumors

Treatment options include:

- Local radiation therapy (RT) and/or skin-directed therapy
- Systemic therapy with or without local RT. Skin-directed therapy might be added. For preferred systemic therapy options, **see Guide 4.**

Widespread tumors

The goal is to reduce the amount of cancer in the body and to prevent further spread.

Treatment options include:

- TSEBT
- Systemic therapy alone or with skin-directed therapy. For preferred systemic therapy options, **see Guide 4.**

Relapse

When cancer returns after a disease-free period, it is called a relapse. Relapse can happen after a complete or partial response to primary treatment. Cancer might be restaged. Depending on the stage, the same or another treatment might be given.

Guide 4
Preferred systemic therapies: Stage 2B

Limited tumors	• Bexarotene • Brentuximab vedotin • Interferon • Methotrexate • Mogamulizumab • Romidepsin
Widespread tumors	• Bexarotene • Brentuximab vedotin • Denileukin diftitox-cxdl • Gemcitabine • Interferon • Liposomal doxorubicin • Methotrexate • Mogamulizumab • Pralatrexate • Romidepsin • Retinoid with interferon

Progression

If cancer spreads or advances to a stage higher than 2B, then the cancer will be restaged. Treatment will be based on the new stage.

Persistent

Persistent is disease that remains after completing primary or main treatment. Treatment is a treatment not used before. The aim is to reduce the amount of cancer before choosing a treatment for refractory disease.

Refractory

When cancer appears resistant to multiple therapies, it is called refractory.

Treatment options include:

- Total skin electron beam therapy (TSEBT)
- Systemic therapy if large cell transformation (LCT). See page 48.
- Other systemic therapies
- Clinical trial
- Allogeneic HCT

An HCT is not an option for everyone. It works best when your lymphoma is responding to therapy. LCT can happen at any stage and is identified by the presence of large cells in a skin or lymph node biopsy.

Stage 3

Stage 3 is also called erythrodermic disease. In erythrodermic disease, nearly all of the skin is reddened (erythema). Cancer may be in lymph nodes (any N) or blood (B1). Treatment is systemic therapy with skin-directed therapy.

Since erythroderma covers most of the body, skin-directed therapies will be for general skin involvement. These include phototherapy, topical corticosteroids, topical mechlorethamine, and total skin electron beam therapy (TSEBT).

For preferred systemic therapy options, **see Guide 5.**

Guide 5 Preferred systemic therapies: Stage 3
Bexarotene
Brentuximab vedotin
Extracorporeal photopheresis (ECP)
Interferon
Methotrexate
Mogamulizumab
Romidepsin
ECP with interferon or retinoid
ECP with interferon and retinoid
Retinoid with interferon

Stage 4

Stage $4A_1$ is Sézary syndrome and is discussed in *Chapter 6: Sézary syndrome.*

Non-Sézary disease (stage 4A2)

In non-Sézary stage 4A2 disease, skin can be any stage (any T). Abnormal T lymphocytes have altered the structure of lymph nodes (N3). Cancer may be found in blood. Treatment is systemic therapy. Radiation therapy might be added to treat skin lesions. A clinical trial or allogeneic hematopoietic cell transplant (HCT) is possible. An HCT is not for everyone. Ask your care team why one treatment might be preferred over another.

Visceral disease (stage 4B)

Visceral disease is cancer that has spread or metastasized to a solid organ such as the spleen or liver. Imaging tests will be used to confirm visceral disease and might be used to see how your body is responding to treatment.

In stage 4B, cancer has metastasized (M1) to internal (visceral) organs or bone marrow. Skin can be any stage (any T). Lymph nodes and blood can be any stage (any N, any B).

Stage 4B disease can occur in mycosis fungoides (MF) or Sézary syndrome (SS). Treatment is systemic therapy alone or with radiation therapy. Systemic therapy works throughout the body to reduce the amount of cancer in the organs and blood. It includes retinoids, chemotherapy, targeted therapy, and immunotherapy. Radiation therapy might be added to treat skin lesions. A clinical trial or allogeneic HCT is possible.

Preferred systemic therapies MF stage 4

- Bexarotene
- Gemcitabine
- Liposomal doxorubicin
- Pralatrexate
- Romidepsin

Large cell transformation

Overview

Large cell transformation (LCT) occurs when a specific group of mycosis fungoides (MF) tumor cells undergo molecular and/or genetic changes that cause them to become larger. LCT can happen at any stage and is identified by the presence of large cells on a skin or lymph node biopsy.

If LCT is suspected, you might have a biopsy. LCT is diagnosed when large cells are present in more than 25 percent (25%) of tumor cells in a skin lesion biopsy. This means that a large cell is found in more than 1 out of every 4 tumor cells. Typically, mycosis fungoides (MF) grows and progresses slowly, but sometimes it transforms in LCT and may become more aggressive. The goal of treatment is to slow the growth of LCT.

Limited lesions with LCT

If there are a limited number of lesions with LCT, the lesions might be treated with radiation therapy (RT).

Widespread lesions with LCT

Treatment options for widespread skin lesions with LCT include total skin electron beam therapy (TSEBT) or systemic therapy with skin-directed therapy. Systemic therapy will help control LCT that is found in any organs and skin lesions. Imaging and other tests might be performed if disease is suspected in lymph nodes and/or internal (visceral) organs.

Preferred systemic therapy options are:

- Brentuximab vedotin
- Gemcitabine
- Liposomal doxorubicin
- Pralatrexate
- Romidepsin
- Systemic therapies for T-cell lymphomas

Relapse

When cancer returns after a disease-free period, it is called a relapse. Treatment might be the same as before, a clinical trial, or allogeneic hematopoietic cell transplant (HCT). Treatment for MF will be based on cancer stage.

Persistent

In LCT that persists, but has not progressed, treatment will focus on reducing the amount of cancer before starting treatment for refractory disease.

Refractory

When cancer appears resistant to multiple therapies, it is called refractory. Treatment might be clinical trial, systemic therapy, or allogeneic HCT.

Key points

- In stage 1A, cancer is limited to a small area on the skin. Less than 10% of the skin (BSA) is covered in patches, papules, and/or plaques. Treatment is skin-directed therapy.
- Treatment for stage 1B and 2A is based on the amount of skin disease.
- Stage 2B is also called tumor stage disease. Treatment is based on if the tumors are limited or widespread.
- Stage 3 is also called erythrodermic disease. In erythrodermic disease, nearly all of the skin is reddened (erythema). Treatment is systemic therapy with skin-directed therapy.
- In stage $4A_2$ disease, abnormal T lymphocytes have altered the structure of lymph nodes (N3). Cancer may be found in blood.
- In stage 4B visceral disease, cancer is found in an internal solid organ such as the spleen or liver, or in the bone marrow.
- Large cell transformation (LCT) can happen at any stage and is identified by the presence of large cells on a skin or lymph node biopsy.

Let us know what you think!

Please take a moment to complete an online survey about the NCCN Guidelines for Patients.

NCCN.org/patients/response

6
Sézary syndrome

In Sézary syndrome (SS), cancerous T cells called Sézary cells may be found in the skin, blood, and lymph nodes. Cancer may be found in a solid, internal organ such as the liver or spleen or in the bone marrow. Treatment is a combination of systemic (drug) therapy with skin-directed therapy. Together, you and your care team will choose a treatment plan that is best for you.

Overview

In Sézary syndrome (SS), a high number of cancerous T cells called Sézary cells are found in the blood. Cancerous T cells may also be found in the skin, lymph nodes, or internal organs. Enlarged lymph nodes (lymphadenopathy) are common. A widespread red rash called erythroderma may cover most of the body.

SS uses the same staging system as mycosis fungoides but is treated differently. SS can be stage $4A_1$, $4A_2$, or 4B. Skin can be any stage (any T). A diagnosis of SS requires B2 blood involvement, which means that a high percentage of Sézary cells are found in the blood. Cancer may be found in bone marrow (M1A) or internal organs (M1B).

Erythroderma

Erythroderma is severe inflammation of most of the body's skin surface. It can look like sunburn or large splotches.

Credit: https://commons.wikimedia.org/wiki/File:Sezery2.jpg

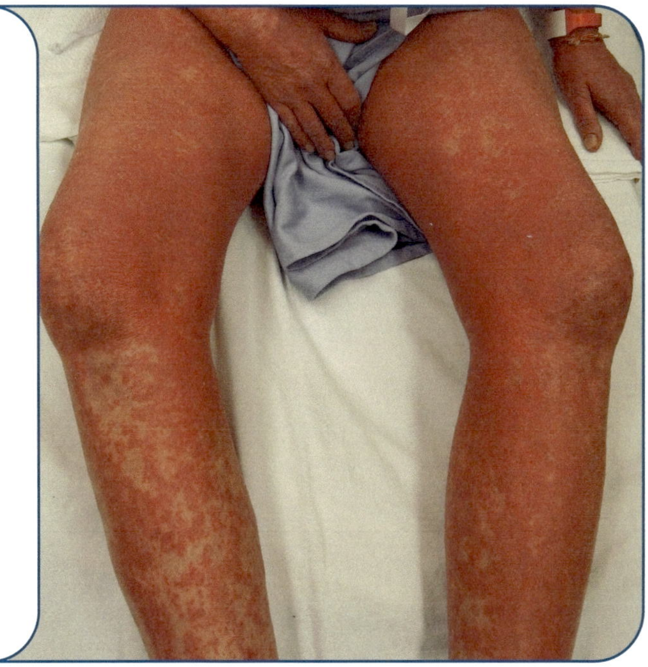

Treatment

Treatment is based on whether disease burden is low or high. Burden refers to the amount of disease in the body. The goal of treatment is to reduce disease burden by combining systemic therapy with skin-directed therapy.

Relapse

When cancer returns after a disease-free period, it is called a relapse. Relapse can happen after a complete or partial response. Treatment is based on disease burden. It might be the same treatment as before or a different one from the list.

Persistent

Persistent disease should be treated with a different systemic therapy than before. The goal is to improve response before moving on to treatment for refractory disease.

Refractory

When cancer appears resistant to multiple therapies, it is called refractory.

Treatment options include:

- Clinical trial
- Systemic therapy. Radiation therapy might be added to treat the skin.
- Allogeneic HCT

An HCT is not for everyone. Ask your care team which option might be best for your type of SS. Your wishes are always important.

Sézary syndrome Preferred drug regimens

Low to intermediate disease burden

- Bexarotene
- Extracorporeal photopheresis (ECP)
- Interferon
- Methotrexate
- Mogamulizumab
- Romidepsin
- Vorinostat
- ECP with interferon or retinoid
- ECP with interferon and retinoid
- Retinoid with interferon

High disease burden

- Mogamulizumab
- Romidepsin
- ECP with interferon or retinoid
- ECP with interferon and retinoid
- Retinoid with interferon

Visceral disease

Visceral disease is stage 4B. It is cancer that has spread or metastasized to a solid, internal organ such as the spleen or liver. Imaging tests are used to confirm visceral disease and might be used to see how your body is responding to treatment.

In stage 4B, cancer has metastasized to the bone marrow (M1A) or to internal (visceral) organs (M1B). Skin can be any stage (any T). Lymph nodes and blood can be any stage (any N, any B). This means cancer may or may not be in the lymph nodes and/or blood.

Both mycosis fungoides (MF) and Sézary syndrome (SS) can be stage 4B visceral disease. Treatment is systemic therapy alone or with radiation therapy. Systemic therapy works throughout the body to reduce the amount of cancer in the organs and blood. It includes retinoids, chemotherapy, targeted therapy, and immunotherapy. Radiation therapy might be used to treat skin lesions.

Key points

- In Sézary syndrome (SS), a high number cancerous T cells called Sézary cells are found in the blood. Cancerous T cells may also be found in the skin, lymph nodes, or internal organs.
- A widespread red rash called erythroderma may cover most of the body. Erythroderma is caused by abnormal T cells called Sézary cells.
- Enlarged lymph nodes (lymphadenopathy) are common.
- Treatment is a combination of systemic (drug) therapy with skin-directed therapy.
- The goal of treatment is to reduce the amount of cancer in the body and to improve your condition.

7

CD30+ PCTLD

In primary cutaneous CD30+ T-cell lymphoproliferative disorders (PCTLDs), T-cell lymphocytes that are CD30-positive (CD30+) grow and cause skin lesions or nodules. Types of PCTLD include cutaneous anaplastic large cell lymphoma (ALCL), lymphomatoid papulosis (LyP), and borderline cases.

Overview

Primary cutaneous CD30+ T-cell lymphoproliferative disorders (PCTLDs) are a group of diseases that include cutaneous anaplastic large cell lymphoma (ALCL), lymphomatoid papulosis (LyP), and borderline cases with overlapping features. In PCTLD, a protein called CD30 is found on the surface of T cells. This is referred to as CD30-posiitve or CD30+. These CD30+ cells grow out of control (proliferate) and cause skin lesions or nodules. Typically, in PCTLD, more than 75 percent (75%) of T cells are CD30+. This means that at least 3 out of every 4 T cells have a protein called CD30 on their surface (CD30+).

Diagnosis aims to distinguish between primary cutaneous anaplastic large cell lymphoma (PC-ALCL) and LyP. Diagnosis is based on the appearance of the lesions and how the disease behaves over time. A skin biopsy might be done.

Types of PCTLDs discussed in this chapter include:

- **Primary cutaneous anaplastic large cell lymphoma (PC-ALCL)** is defined by the presence of anaplastic large cells. Lesions appear on the skin as one or more raised, red lesions or nodules. Anaplastic cells are fast-growing, abnormal cells. PC-ALCL starts in the skin and may spread to the lymph nodes.
- **Lymphomatoid papulosis (LyP)** is a benign, chronic, recurring, self-healing condition. Papulonodular skin lesions appear on the skin as small bumps and nodules.

In addition, a person can have both PCTLD and mycosis fungoides (MF). MF or Sézary syndrome (SS) that is CD30+ is not the same as PCTLD. Sézary cells are typically CD30-.

Primary cutaneous ALCL

Anaplastic large cell lymphoma (ALCL) can be found in the skin, the lymph nodes, or in organs throughout the body. When ALCL appears in the skin, it is called primary cutaneous ALCL (PC-ALCL) or cutaneous ALCL. PC-ALCL may also be found in a nearby (regional) lymph node. Sometimes, cutaneous ALCL can extend beyond the skin and lymph nodes to organs. If this occurs, it is usually treated as systemic ALCL.

For treatment of systemic ALCL, see *NCCN Guidelines for Patients: Peripheral T-Cell Lymphoma* at NCCN.org/patientguidelines and on the NCCN Patient Guides for Cancer app.

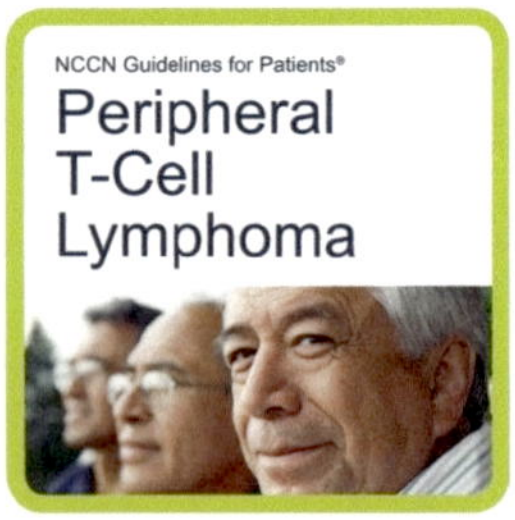

Treatment

PC-ALCL is often a slowing-growing (indolent), persistent disease with lesions that may go away (regress). Lesions often return but seem to respond well to treatment. Not everyone's disease responds to treatment the same way. Treatment for PC-ALCL is based on the number of lesions and their location.

One or grouped lesions

Primary treatment is the first treatment. Treatment aims to remove the lesion. This can be achieved using involved-site radiation therapy (ISRT), surgery (excision), or both. ISRT is more common.

After a response to treatment, you will be monitored for recurrence. Recurrence or relapse is the return of one or more lesions. If a lesion returns and is confined to the skin, then you can be retreated with ISRT, surgery, or both. Sometimes, observation (no treatment) is an option if the lesions are not causing symptoms (asymptomatic). If no response or lesions seem resistant (refractory) to treatment, then you will be treated as described below in multifocal lesions.

Multifocal lesions

When there are lesions in multiple locations, primary treatment focuses on systemic therapy such as brentuximab vedotin (Adcetris). Other systemic therapies might be given alone or with skin-directed therapy.

After a response to treatment, you will be observed for recurrence. Recurrence or relapse is the return of multifocal lesions. If relapse, no response, or lesions seem resistant (refractory) to treatment, then options include:

- Clinical trial
- Same treatment as before (unless refractory or intolerant)
- Different treatment from before

- Other systemic therapies such as those found under large cell transformation in *Chapter 6: Mycosis fungoides*

PC-ALCL with regional lymph node involvement

PC-ALCL may involve the skin and nearby (regional) lymph nodes. A lymph node biopsy is needed to confirm disease. Treatment aims to reduce the amount of skin lesions and disease in lymph nodes. The preferred treatment is brentuximab vedotin (Adcetris) with or without involved-site radiation therapy (ISRT) to lymph nodes and primary skin lesions. Other systemic therapies might be given.

After a response to treatment, you will be observed for recurrence. Recurrence or relapse is the return of disease. If relapse, no response, or lesions seem resistant (refractory) to treatment, then options include:

- Clinical trial
- Same treatment as before (unless refractory or intolerant)
- Different treatment from before
- Other systemic therapies such as those found under large cell transformation in *Chapter 6: Mycosis fungoides*

LyP

Lymphomatoid papulosis (LyP) is a benign, chronic, recurring disease of the immune system. Lesions appear on the skin as small bumps and nodules called papulonodular skin lesions. LyP is a primary cutaneous CD30+ T-cell lymphoproliferative disorder (PCTLD). Lymphoproliferative disorders are often treated like cancer, but they are not cancer.

Your preferences about treatment are always important. If you have any religious or personal beliefs about certain kinds of treatment, share them with your care team and make your wishes known.

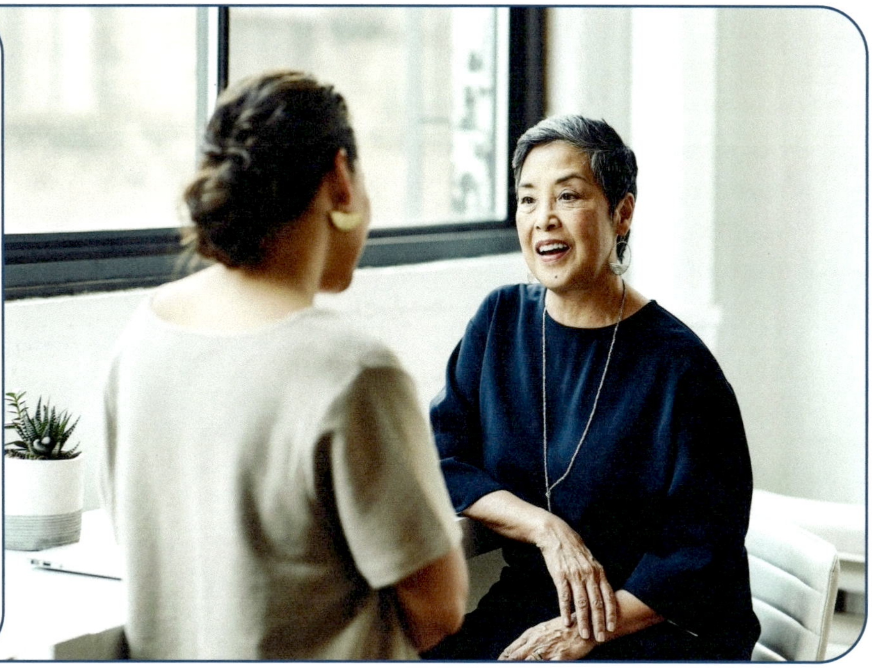

Treatment for limited lesions

- **Without symptoms** – An asymptomatic person is without symptoms. Observation is the preferred option for those with limited lesions who are asymptomatic. Topical steroids are also an option.
- **With symptoms** – If you have limited lesions with symptoms, treatment aims to reduce symptoms. Topical steroids and phototherapy are common. Observation is also an option.
- **If disease is responding to treatment**, then you will continue the same treatment.
- **If no response or refractory disease,** then the options are a different treatment or clinical trial.

Treatment for widespread lesions

Treatment for widespread lesions aims to reduce the number of lesions and any discomfort they may cause. This may be done using skin-directed or systemic therapies. Observation is preferred for those without symptoms (asymptomatic).

- **If disease is responding to treatment,** then you will be observed for recurrence. Recurrence or relapse is the return of disease.
- **For relapse,** options are a clinical trial, observation, same treatment as before, or different treatment from before.
- **If no response or refractory disease,** then the options are a treatment not used before, brentuximab vedotin, or clinical trial. When cancer appears resistant to multiple therapies, it is called refractory.

Monitoring

Those with LyP are at risk for developing another type of lymphoma. Life-long follow-up will be needed. Your doctor should conduct a thorough skin exam during each follow-up visit. Ask how you will be monitored and how often you should have a check-up.

Key points

- In primary cutaneous CD30+ T-cell lymphoproliferative disorders (PCTLDs), T-cell lymphocytes that are CD30-positive (CD30+) grow and cause skin lesions or nodules.
- Types of PCTLD include cutaneous anaplastic large cell lymphoma (ALCL), lymphomatoid papulosis (LyP), and borderline cases.
- Diagnosis aims to distinguish between cutaneous ALCL and LyP.
- Cutaneous ALCL appears in the skin as one or more raised lesions or nodules and may be found in lymph nodes.
- LyP is a benign (not cancer), chronic, recurring disease of the immune system.
- Treatment for LyP includes skin-directed and/or systemic therapy. A clinical trial may be an option.
- A person can have both PCTLD and mycosis fungoides (MF).

8

Making treatment decisions

It's important to be comfortable with the cancer treatment you choose. This choice starts with having an open and honest conversation with your care team.

It's your choice

In shared decision-making, you and your care team share information, discuss the options, and agree on a treatment plan. It starts with an open and honest conversation between you and your care team.

Treatment decisions are very personal. What is important to you may not be important to someone else. Some things that may play a role in your decision-making:

- What you want and how that might differ from what others want
- Your religious and spiritual beliefs
- Your feelings about certain treatments
- Your feelings about pain or side effects
- Cost of treatment, travel to treatment centers, and time away from school or work
- Quality of life and length of life
- How active you are and the activities that are important to you

Think about what you want from treatment. Discuss openly the risks and benefits of specific treatments and procedures. Weigh options and share concerns with your care team. If you take the time to build a relationship with your care team, it will help you feel supported when considering options and making treatment decisions.

Second opinion

It is normal to want to start treatment as soon as possible. While cancer can't be ignored, there is time to have another doctor review your test results and suggest a treatment plan. This is called getting a second opinion, and it's a normal part of cancer care. Even doctors get second opinions!

Things you can do to prepare:

- Check with your insurance company about its rules on second opinions. There may be out-of-pocket costs to see doctors who are not part of your insurance plan.
- Make plans to have copies of all your records sent to the doctor you will see for your second opinion.

Support groups

Many people diagnosed with cancer find support groups to be helpful. Support groups often include people at different stages of treatment. Some people may be newly diagnosed, while others may be finished with treatment. If your hospital or community doesn't have support groups for people with cancer, check out the websites listed in this book.

Questions to ask

Possible questions to ask your care team are listed on the following pages. Feel free to use these questions or come up with your own.

Questions about testing and diagnosis

1. What type of cancer do I have? What does this mean in terms of my prognosis and treatment options?
2. Is cancer in my blood, lymph nodes, or other organs?
3. Is there a cancer center or hospital nearby that specializes in this type of cancer?
4. What tests will I have? How often will they be repeated?
5. Will my insurance pay for this test?
6. When will I know the test results and who will explain them to me?
7. Would you give me a copy of the pathology report and other test results?
8. Who will talk with me about the next steps? When?
9. Will treatment start before the test results are in?

Questions about skin

1. Can I use lotions or oils on my skin or hair other than what you give me? What are the best types of soap, shampoo, sunscreen, hair dye, or makeup for me to use?

2. Is it better to wear long sleeves or pants, or to cover the rash/lesions in some way? Or should I let my skin be exposed to the air as much as possible?

3. Should I take time to inspect my skin? If so, how often?

4. If I notice any changes in my skin whom should I call and when?

5. Will keeping a diary and photo journal help? What should I include in the diary? How often should I take photos?

6. Can I go out in the sun? Should I wear sunscreen, long sleeves, or a hat?

7. Are there any changes that I can make to my diet, or activity and stress level that will help my condition?

Questions about your care team's experience

1. What is your experience treating this type of cancer?
2. What is the experience of those on your team?
3. What types of cancer do you treat?
4. I would like to get a second opinion. Is there someone you recommend?
5. How many people like me (of the same age, gender, race) have you treated?
6. Will you be consulting with experts to discuss my care? Whom will you consult?
7. How many procedures like the one you're suggesting have you done?
8. Is this treatment a major part of your practice?
9. What types of complications are possible?
10. Who will manage my day-to-day care?

Questions about options

1. What will happen if I do nothing?
2. Am I a candidate for a clinical trial?
3. Can I join a clinical trial at any time?
4. Which option is proven to work best for my cancer, age, overall health, and other factors?
5. What if I am pregnant or am planning to get pregnant soon?
6. Should I see a fertility specialist or genetic counselor?
7. Can I stop treatment at any time? What will happen if I stop treatment?
8. What are my options if treatment doesn't work as expected?
9. What decisions must be made today? Is there a social worker or someone who can help me decide about treatment?
10. Is there a hospital or treatment center you can recommend for treatment?

Questions about treatment

1. Which treatment(s) do you recommend and why?
2. Does this treatment offer a cure? If not, how well can treatment stop the cancer from growing?
3. Does the order of treatment matter?
4. When will I start treatment and how long will treatment likely take?
5. What should I expect from treatment?
6. What will you do to make me comfortable during treatment?
7. How much will my insurance pay for treatment?
8. Are there programs to help me pay for treatment?
9. What are the chances my cancer will return?
10. What is my risk for developing another kind of cancer, such as skin cancer?

Questions about radiation therapy

1. What type of radiation therapy (RT) will I have?
2. What will you target?
3. What is the goal of this radiation treatment?
4. Will RT be used with other therapies?
5. How many treatment sessions will I require?
6. Do you offer this type of radiation here? If not, can you refer me to someone who does?
7. What side effects can I expect from RT?
8. Will I be given medicine to help me relax during RT?
9. What should I wear?

Questions about clinical trials

1. What clinical trials are available for my type and stage of cancer?
2. What are the treatments used in the clinical trial?
3. What does the treatment do?
4. Has the treatment been used before? Has it been used for other types of cancer?
5. What are the risks and benefits of this treatment?
6. What side effects should I expect? How will the side effects be controlled?
7. How long will I be in the clinical trial?
8. Will I be able to get other treatments if this doesn't work?
9. How will you know the treatment is working?
10. Will the clinical trial cost me anything? If so, how much?

Questions about side effects

1. What are the side effects of this treatment?
2. How long will these side effects last?
3. Do any side effects lessen or worsen in severity over time?
4. What side effects are expected and which are life threatening?
5. When should I call the doctor? Can I text?
6. What should I do for an issue on weekends and other non-office hours?
7. What medicines can I take to prevent or relieve side effects?
8. Will you stop treatment or change treatment if there are side effects? What do you look for?
9. What can I do to lessen or prevent side effects? What will you do?
10. What side effects are life-long and irreversible even after completing treatment?

Questions about resources and support

1. Who can I talk to about help with housing, food, and other basic needs?
2. What help is available for transportation, childcare, and home care?
3. How much will I have to pay for treatment?
4. What help is available to pay for medicines and other treatment?
5. What other services are available to me and my caregivers?
6. How can I connect with others and build a support system?
7. How can I find in-person or online support?
8. Who can help me with my concerns about missing work or school?
9. Who can I talk to if I don't feel safe at home, at work, or in my neighborhood?
10. How can I get help to stop smoking or vaping?

Resources

Cancer*Care*
Cancercare.org

Cutaneous Lymphoma Foundation
Clfoundation.org

Imerman Angels
Imermanangels.org

MedlinePlus
medlineplus.gov

National Cancer Institute (NCI)
cancer.gov/types/lymphoma/patient/mycosis-fungoides-treatment-pdq

National Coalition for Cancer Survivorship
canceradvocacy.org

The Leukemia & Lymphoma Society
LLS.org/PatientSupport

Triage Cancer
Triagecancer.org

Words to know

anaplastic
Cancer cells that divide rapidly and do not look like normal cells.

biopsy
The removal of a sample of tissue for testing.

blood tumor burden
The amount of cancerous cells in the blood.

chemotherapy
Drugs that kill fast-growing cells, including cancer cells and normal cells.

clinical trial
A type of research that assesses health tests or treatments.

complete blood count (CBC)
A lab test that includes the number of blood cells.

dermatologist
A doctor who specializes in the diagnosis and treatment of skin diseases.

external beam radiation therapy (EBRT)
A cancer treatment with radiation received from a machine outside the body.

gene
Coded instructions in cells for making new cells and controlling how cells behave.

histology
The structure of cells, tissue, and organs as viewed under a microscope.

imaging test
A test that makes pictures (images) of the insides of the body.

immune system
The body's natural defense against infection and disease.

immunohistochemistry (IHC)
A lab test of cancer cells to find specific cell traits involved in abnormal cell growth.

involved-site radiation therapy (ISRT)
Targets a specific area of skin. It can also be used to treat specific lymph nodes with cancer.

lymph
A clear fluid containing white blood cells.

lymphadenopathy
Lymph nodes that are abnormal in size or consistency.

lymphatic system
Germ-fighting network of tissues and organs that includes the bone marrow, spleen, thymus, lymph nodes, and lymphatic vessels. Part of the immune system.

lymph node
A small, bean-shaped, disease-fighting structure.

medical oncologist
A doctor who is an expert in cancer drugs.

palpable adenopathy
Lymph nodes that feel abnormal in size or consistency.

papule
A small, solid, raised bump on the skin that might look like small pimples. Papules may be red, purple, brown, or pink.

papulonodular
Combination of papules and nodules found on the skin.

patch
A flat, thin, pink or red skin lesion of any size.

pathologist
A doctor who is an expert in testing cells and tissue to find disease.

persistent
Cancer that remains or returns.

phototherapy
Uses different ultraviolet (UV) light wavelengths to treat skin lesions or tumors.

plaque
A raised (elevated) or hardened (indurated) skin lesion of any size.

progression
The growth or spread of cancer after being tested or treated.

radiation therapy (RT)
A treatment that uses high-energy rays or related approaches to kill cancer cells.

refractory
Cancer that does not respond to multiple treatments.

regression
A decrease in the size of a patch, plaque, or tumor or the amount of cancer in the body.

relapse
The return or worsening of cancer after a period of improvement.

remission
There are minor or no signs of disease.

retinoids
Products related to vitamin A.

scale
When the outer layer of skin peels away in large pieces.

side effect
An unhealthy or unpleasant physical or emotional response to treatment.

skin-directed therapy
Treatment focused on the skin. Includes topical therapy, local radiation, and phototherapy.

skin disease burden
The amount of cancerous cells found in the skin.

supportive care
Health care that includes symptom relief but not cancer treatment. Also called palliative care or best supportive care.

systemic therapy
Treatment that works throughout the body.

targeted therapy
A drug treatment that targets and attacks specific cancer cells.

total skin electron beam therapy (TSEBT)
Treats the entire skin surface.

NCCN Contributors

This patient guide is based on the NCCN Clinical Practice Guidelines in Oncology (NCCN Guidelines®) for Primary Cutaneous Lymphomas Version 3.2024 It was adapted, reviewed, and published with help from the following people:

Dorothy A. Shead, MS
Senior Director
Patient Information Operations

Tanya Fischer, MEd, MSLIS
Senior Medical Writer

Laura Phillips
Graphic Artist

The NCCN Clinical Practice Guidelines in Oncology (NCCN Guidelines®) for Primary Cutaneous Lymphomas Version 3.2024 were developed by the following NCCN Panel Members:

Steven M. Horwitz, MD/Chair
Memorial Sloan Kettering Cancer Center

Stephen Ansell, MD, PhD/Vice-Chair
Mayo Clinic Comprehensive Cancer Center

Weiyun Z. Ai, MD, PhD
UCSF Helen Diller Family Comprehensive Cancer Center

Jeffrey Barnes, MD, PhD
Mass General Cancer Center

Stefan K. Barta, MD, MRCP, MS
Abramson Cancer Center at the University of Pennsylvania

Jonathan Brammer, MD
The Ohio State University Comprehensive Cancer Center - James Cancer Hospital and Solove Research Institute

Mark W. Clemens, MD
The University of Texas MD Anderson Cancer Center

Utpal P. Davé, MD
Indiana University Melvin and Bren Simon Comprehensive Cancer Center

Ahmet Dogan, MD, PhD
Memorial Sloan Kettering Cancer Center

Francine Foss, MD
Yale Cancer Center/Smilow Cancer Hospital

Zachary Frosch, MD, MSHP
Fox Chase Cancer Center

Aaron M. Goodman, MD
UC San Diego Moores Cancer Center

Joan Guitart, MD
Robert H. Lurie Comprehensive Cancer Center of Northwestern University

Ahmad Halwani, MD
Huntsman Cancer Institute at the University of Utah

Bradley M. Haverkos, MD, MPH, MS
University of Colorado Cancer Center

Francisco Hernandez-Ilizaliturri, MD
Roswell Park Comprehensive Cancer Center

Richard T. Hoppe, MD
Stanford Cancer Institute

Eric Jacobsen, MD
Dana-Farber/Brigham and Women's Cancer Center

Deepa Jagadeesh, MD, MPH
Case Comprehensive Cancer Center/ University Hospitals Seidman Cancer Center and Cleveland Clinic Taussig Cancer Institute

Allison Jones, MD
St. Jude Children's Research Hospital/ The University of Tennessee Health Science Center

Youn H. Kim, MD
Stanford Cancer Institute

Kiran Kumar, MD, MBA
UT Southwestern Simmons Comprehensive Cancer Center

*Neha Mehta-Shah, MD, MSCI
Siteman Cancer Center at Barnes-Jewish Hospital and Washington University School of Medicine

Elise A. Olsen, MD
Duke Cancer Institute

Saurabh A. Rajguru, MD
University of Wisconsin Carbone Cancer Center

Peter Riedell, MD
The UChicago Medicine Comprehensive Cancer Center

Sima Rozati, MD, PhD
Johns Hopkins Kimmel Cancer Center

Jonathan Said, MD
UCLA Jonsson Comprehensive Cancer Center

Aaron Shaver, MD, PhD
Vanderbilt-Ingram Cancer Center

*Lauren Shea, MD
O'Neal Comprehensive Cancer Center at UAB

*Michi M. Shinohara, MD
Fred Hutchinson Cancer Center

Lubomir Sokol, MD, PhD
Moffitt Cancer Center

Matthew Stephany, MD
Fred & Pamela Buffett Cancer Center

*Susan Thornton
Patient Advocate

*Carlos Torres-Cabala, MD
The University of Texas MD Anderson Cancer Center

Ryan Wilcox, MD, PhD
University of Michigan Rogel Cancer Center

Peggy Wu, MD, MPH
UC Davis Comprehensive Cancer Center

Jasmine Zain, MD
City of Hope National Medical Center

NCCN

Mary Dwyer, MS
Senior Director, Guidelines Operations

Hema Sundar, PhD
Senior Manager, Global Clinical Content

* Reviewed this patient guide. For disclosures, visit NCCN.org/disclosures.

NCCN Cancer Centers

Abramson Cancer Center
at the University of Pennsylvania
Philadelphia, Pennsylvania
800.789.7366 • pennmedicine.org/cancer

Case Comprehensive Cancer Center/
University Hospitals Seidman Cancer Center and
Cleveland Clinic Taussig Cancer Institute
Cleveland, Ohio
UH Seidman Cancer Center
800.641.2422 • uhhospitals.org/services/cancer-services
CC Taussig Cancer Institute
866.223.8100 • my.clevelandclinic.org/departments/cancer
Case CCC
216.844.8797 • case.edu/cancer

City of Hope National Medical Center
Duarte, California
800.826.4673 • cityofhope.org

Dana-Farber/Brigham and Women's Cancer Center |
Mass General Cancer Center
Boston, Massachusetts
877.442.3324 • youhaveus.org
617.726.5130 • massgeneral.org/cancer-center

Duke Cancer Institute
Durham, North Carolina
888.275.3853 • dukecancerinstitute.org

Fox Chase Cancer Center
Philadelphia, Pennsylvania
888.369.2427 • foxchase.org

Fred & Pamela Buffett Cancer Center
Omaha, Nebraska
402.559.5600 • unmc.edu/cancercenter

Fred Hutchinson Cancer Center
Seattle, Washington
206.667.5000 • fredhutch.org

Huntsman Cancer Institute at the University of Utah
Salt Lake City, Utah
800.824.2073 • healthcare.utah.edu/huntsmancancerinstitute

Indiana University Melvin and Bren Simon
Comprehensive Cancer Center
Indianapolis, Indiana
888.600.4822 • www.cancer.iu.edu

Johns Hopkins Kimmel Cancer Center
Baltimore, Maryland
410.955.8964
www.hopkinskimmelcancercenter.org

Mayo Clinic Comprehensive Cancer Center
Phoenix/Scottsdale, Arizona
Jacksonville, Florida
Rochester, Minnesota
480.301.8000 • Arizona
904.953.0853 • Florida
507.538.3270 • Minnesota
mayoclinic.org/cancercenter

Memorial Sloan Kettering Cancer Center
New York, New York
800.525.2225 • mskcc.org

Moffitt Cancer Center
Tampa, Florida
888.663.3488 • moffitt.org

O'Neal Comprehensive Cancer Center at UAB
Birmingham, Alabama
800.822.0933 • uab.edu/onealcancercenter

Robert H. Lurie Comprehensive Cancer Center
of Northwestern University
Chicago, Illinois
866.587.4322 • cancer.northwestern.edu

Roswell Park Comprehensive Cancer Center
Buffalo, New York
877.275.7724 • roswellpark.org

Siteman Cancer Center at Barnes-Jewish Hospital
and Washington University School of Medicine
St. Louis, Missouri
800.600.3606 • siteman.wustl.edu

St. Jude Children's Research Hospital/
The University of Tennessee Health Science Center
Memphis, Tennessee
866.278.5833 • stjude.org
901.448.5500 • uthsc.edu

Stanford Cancer Institute
Stanford, California
877.668.7535 • cancer.stanford.edu

The Ohio State University Comprehensive Cancer Center -
James Cancer Hospital and Solove Research Institute
Columbus, Ohio
800.293.5066 • cancer.osu.edu

The UChicago Medicine Comprehensive Cancer Center
Chicago, Illinois
773.702.1000 • uchicagomedicine.org/cancer

The University of Texas MD Anderson Cancer Center
Houston, Texas
844.269.5922 • mdanderson.org

UC Davis Comprehensive Cancer Center
Sacramento, California
916.734.5959 • 800.770.9261
health.ucdavis.edu/cancer

UC San Diego Moores Cancer Center
La Jolla, California
858.822.6100 • cancer.ucsd.edu

UCLA Jonsson Comprehensive Cancer Center
Los Angeles, California
310.825.5268 • uclahealth.org/cancer

UCSF Helen Diller Family
Comprehensive Cancer Center
San Francisco, California
800.689.8273 • cancer.ucsf.edu

University of Colorado Cancer Center
Aurora, Colorado
720.848.0300 • coloradocancercenter.org

University of Michigan Rogel Cancer Center
Ann Arbor, Michigan
800.865.1125 • rogelcancercenter.org

University of Wisconsin Carbone Cancer Center
Madison, Wisconsin
608.265.1700 • uwhealth.org/cancer

UT Southwestern Simmons
Comprehensive Cancer Center
Dallas, Texas
214.648.3111 • utsouthwestern.edu/simmons

Vanderbilt-Ingram Cancer Center
Nashville, Tennessee
877.936.8422 • vicc.org

Yale Cancer Center/Smilow Cancer Hospital
New Haven, Connecticut
855.4.SMILOW • yalecancercenter.org

share with us.

Take our survey and help make the NCCN Guidelines for Patients better for everyone!

NCCN.org/patients/comments

Notes

Index

Made in the USA
Monee, IL
12 September 2026

62980079R00048